BOOK V

DECODING SEXUALITY AND SPIRITUALITY

A METAPHYSICAL INTERPRETATION

O.M. KELLY

COPYRIGHT

AUTHOR

Author O. M. Kelly, known as Omni to her clients and students is an accomplished author and international lecturer, on Metaphysics, Philosophy and understanding the Collective Consciousness. Omni consults for Member States of the European Commission as a Conciliation Advisor and Rhetoric Counsellor for other International Companies throughout Europe. Omni now resides on Australia's beautiful Gold Coast, writing books, and works as a Life Mentor and Business Coach.

Omni has dedicated her life to decoding the mysteries of the universe. With a deep knowledge of the biblical agenda, mythologies including ancient Egyptology, Asian principles, and metaphysical insights, Omni has discovered the secret that all stories share a coded hidden metaphysical language. Her seminal work, "Decoding the Mind of God", is a compilation of nine volumes of metaphysical information based on the research into the coded information of the Laws of the Universe, also known as the Collective Consciousness, and represents a groundbreaking contribution to our understanding of the metaphysical universe. Now, all nine volumes are being released as separate, revised books, each offering a unique perspective on the universe's workings. Omni's work has been widely acclaimed for its depth of insight, and her contributions to the field of metaphysics have been groundbreaking.

THIS BOOK

Unlock the mysteries of sexuality and spirituality with "Decoding Sexuality and Spirituality: A Metaphysical Interpretation" by O.M. Kelly (Omni). This groundbreaking book offers a fresh perspective on the ways in which our sexuality and spirituality intersect and influence each other.

This book explores a wide range of topics related to sexuality and spirituality, including the idea that sexuality is the doorway to our spirituality. It also delves into the Testament of the Oracle, the orgasmic cloud, and the role of marriage in our sexual and spiritual lives.

Readers will be inspired to contemplate the decision to conceive or not conceive, and gain a deeper understanding of the journey as a woman. They will also explore the importance of timing when it comes to sex and the ways in which our sexuality can manipulate our spirituality.

Drawing on deep knowledge of the biblical agenda, mythologies, including Egyptology, and metaphysical insights, Omni has discovered the codes hidden in the metaphysical language that relate to the unlocking the true potential of our sexual and spiritual lives.

So, whether you are seeking to deepen your understanding of sexuality and spirituality, or simply looking for a new perspective on these important topics, "Decoding Sexuality and Spirituality" is the book for you. Start your journey towards a more fulfilling, meaningful life.

CONTENTS

Introduction

INTRODUCTION

In this book, we will explore the fascinating relationship between our sexuality and spirituality, and how these two aspects of ourselves are intimately intertwined. This book explains the importance of sexuality in our daily lives, and it is explained in a manner of concise information. We must understand that hidden codes relating to our sexual behaviour are lying enveloped in our DNA, and they are brought forward into our life through our past generations' fear of themselves.

Once we have accepted this fact, we find that it releases the pressure of self; we start to open up our cellular bodies, where we are led into the discovery of the embedded intelligence released through one's self-worth. It is here that we first bring to our attention the negative thinking of the mind overriding its possibilities. As we become aware of this trapped energy, we begin to move forward and fight our way out of this inertia. The extreme force we find within is where our sexual prowess begins to come alive.

This gives us the opportunity to go forth and release our sexual freedom through understanding the first basic level of humanity's intelligence.
Omni

"Woman becomes the comfort zone for man, where he can rest and find a home for the compatibility of his ego, preferably without restraint. He then has the opportunity to release his tension, which allows him to socialize back into his emotional self, and the nourishment that woman receives becomes the contentment she is striving so hard to achieve. It is the basic evolution of our life yearning to achieve its own self-satisfaction."
Omni

CHAPTER ONE

Sexuality Is The Doorway To Our Spirituality

The hieroglyphs in Egypt explain the stories of the Metaphysical language of man. These Semitic sounds were collected and rephrased and written by the hierarchical mind – and they were collected from the early Akkadian, through to the Aramaic translation, and through to the ancient Egyptian empire. As they were brought into the Greek philosophies, these same stories were released and brought up into the ancient Asiatic principles through the Book of Revelations, in order to be exemplified, and all of them were placed in the Holy Bible.

This book was, and is, a teaching tool for the highest order of the religious experience we have chosen to live by; it explains to us the secrets to the importance of the Hidden God. This Hidden God is embedded in every cell in the human body; it is the light of intelligence that all these stories relate to; it is every myth that has been spoken and transferred down through the generations – from the most ancient to modern-day man. These stories are also from every religion that man has created for the satisfaction of balancing his own ego. If we can accept credit for those stories, we can also realize and accept that they were placed here as a guideline for us to understand that our sexuality is the doorway to our Spirituality. We are not born from any other section of the body; we manifest in the womb and mostly birth through the vagina. (Surgeries and IVF procedures notwithstanding, this is still the most typical.)

Remember, those hidden codes relating to our sexual behaviour are lying enveloped in our DNA, and we have innocently buried that behaviour beneath the layers of our own confinement, through our not being aware of how to understand our fear. That fear has been brought forward into our life through our past generations' fear of attending to themselves. Once we can understand and accept this, it will then give us the opportunity to release our sexual freedom, through searching for the answers and releasing them to our inner selves.

Our journey is to contact the Hidden God that is within us all. Through understanding and accepting this information, we are given the opportunity to walk forward in confidence through the maze of life's expectancies. All of which releases the pressure of self, where we begin to open up our cellular light – or intellectual bodies – which leads us into discovering our intelligence regarding our own self-worth.

It is when we innocently fear ourselves through how and what we think, that we first bring to our own attention the sexual molestation of the mind overriding its possibilities! When we live in fear of what is expected of us, our innocence becomes trapped. Through that building upon itself, our fear then climbs up and sits on top of us, searching for security, and it chokes off our understanding of self-growth. As we become aware of that trapped energy, we begin to move forward and fight our way out of that old inertia that we have innocently allowed to take hold. This fight is created through our sexual impatience, which can become an extreme force that we awaken within us. In other words, our sexual prowess comes alive.

Every myth explains its stories to us by way of parables, and, as we are born onto this planet, so, too, does our journey of understanding the Divine within begin in the same way. Our initial understanding of the Adamic principles is explained in exactly the same way.

A man cannot find his freedom of mind until he births the power of his penis, and a woman cannot find her fulfilment until she finds the strength of her clitoris. Let us decipher the word "clitoris". Is it "Kha-EL-it-of-Horus" or "Kha-EL-it-UR-Is"? Which explanation do you think is right, or are they both right? One word is just an extended parasite of the other. Remember that the clitoris is the penis of the woman, and the word "woman" interprets as the "Womb of AN".

We can now understand a little more as to how woman connects to the emotional worlds of the second stage of us becoming as God is when she moves into a relationship with another being. If man is from the first God – which, through the myth we have named "EL" – and woman is from the second God – which we now know as "AN" – then we can accept the reasoning as to why we need the relationship of a "sexu-EL" experience, with them both attracted to one another. Man is there to nourish; and woman becomes the nurturer. Of course, this attracts the light and brief state of enlightenment that autonomically collects as the nervous system is stimulated through copulation, which creates both orgasm and ejaculation – or sexual fulfilment.

Woman becomes the comfort zone for man, where he can rest and find a home for the compatibility of his ego, preferably without restraint. He then has the opportunity to release his tension, which allows him to socialize back into his emotional self, and the nourishment that woman receives becomes the contentment she is striving so hard to achieve. It is the basic evolution of our life yearning to achieve its own self-satisfaction.

Your Notes:

CHAPTER TWO

The Testament Of The Oracle

Come with me now, and I will tell you another story. At one time, there was a King or Pharaoh whose name was "Tut-Mose". When we go back into the ancient wisdom, we find that it is the quest of the Pharaoh's life to birth himself, to come into discovering the capabilities of his own mind – which, at that time, was through his subjects devoting their life to him, rather than through him relying on himself.

While he had others to do his bidding, he escaped the laws of Karma, and he was also innocent to the laws of his own Oracle, which was his Inner Universe at that time (Law of Self). The origins of the story began to be passed onto us through it being carved onto the walls of the temples in Egypt. He had himself totally under his own control, and he could not bend or sway in order to allow himself to release his own emotional intelligence. He used only his left brain, so there was no freedom in his mind – there was no yearning, learning, or earning, and this became the introduction of us being introduced into the mythical quest.

He had only one word in his dictionary: "control", and this word means "to be conned by the Troll". The Troll is embedded within each of us, and it represents the animal primordial mind of our past evolution that has come along for the ride with each and every one of us. It is the basic foundation of the creation of our DNA. Some call it the "devil"; others refer to it as the "dragon within"; still others refer to it as the "beast".

The name Tut-Mose (through Moses understanding that his truth as he knew it to be, was learning to understand his inner truth) was rearranged for the stories in the Bible. It began with the name Mosea, where we learn to "master the Oracle of our Soul to 'EA'". As time moved on, it was intellectualized, and later transcribed as Moses, which explains to us the plural mind of humanity. We slowly advanced into the word, which also coincides with the word "Moschee" in the ancient language, through to the language of the Romans (i.e., Latin), which referred to it as "Moschea". In the English language, this word is pronounced as "Mosque", which we now are fully aware of as the Muslim place of worship.

I would like to explain to you how the story was brought down to us through the Metaphysical language, where we began to understand and create the stories of Moses leading his people to the Promised Land. It was only when I went to Europe, years after my journey had completed itself, that all my years of research to bring my intelligence up through the evolution of humanity could explain my truth to me. I had held this sacred information in regard to myself for many years, waiting in anticipation for the reflection of what I had learned and earned to be mirrored and returned back to me.

Through the German language, the word for the prepuce is the introduction into circumcision, and it is called the "phimose" – or "the balance of Moses". The prepuce is where the foreskin connects under the tip of the penis. When that prepuce is cut and removed, the penis is free to release the collection of its own restrictions; these restrictions have been created through the collection of the fear that was held back in the previous generations. The penis has evolved in that way to remind the male species that the ego, which is controlled through the energy of the penis (individually and collectively), cannot be forced. It can be urged, and an urge comes from the inner strength one is collecting through the action of respecting others, and receiving for one's self. It is the first step to discovering our God within. Remember that there are three worlds that we live in, and, as we leave one world, we are brought up into the next one. Hence, the explanation of the three-dimensional mind, which is represented by the names of the three Gods: "EL", "AN", "EA". Interpreted through the matter of physics – or the Metaphysical language – these three names are here to remind us that we can attain Everlasting Life, Ascending and Nourishing, with an Energetic Attitude. All this is similar to how we introduced our self into our spoken word, which was released to us through our DNA. Always remember, the first step is the hardest!

When man tries to overemphasize his own strength, God

steps in to remind him that he is stepping outside his own intellectual boundaries; especially when he has not yet earned his next evolutionary step. We must remember, too, that the penis is the first kingdom we overcome on the way to educating ourselves. Once we are educated, we learn how to open our heart, where the penis energy comes up through the heart to relate to others – that is, it is how it earns its second step. The penis energy is transformed through the opening of the heart, up into the tongue, where both begin to relate with one another through being connected to both the upper and lower kingdoms of Egypt.

During the days in my clinic when many of you walked in the door to be heard, I noticed that the fear in some of the men had placed a strangle hold around their penis. They came in with this choking feeling around the sexual area. This irritation caused rashes, itches, blisters, etc. – even to the point where they had difficulty holding onto their urine. When we went back into their childhood, they could begin to accept that their thoughts were strangled, which was caused mainly through an overbearing father. These men did not have the confidence in themselves to speak their truth, so they began to stutter their words. The thoughts that they wanted to speak were held back, and they had difficulty finding a way to release themselves. Their inner dictionary became scrambled, and, as they tried to speak their mind, their ego stepped in to regain control over their thoughts. Once we could acknowledge the story behind the strangulation, the stuttering of their words miraculously disappeared.

The Old Testament of the Bible, in the Book of Exodus, begins to explain the story of man awakening to himself from an inner level, and it seems it all began with the creation of Moses. Moses went out into the desert for forty years, searching for his freedom, and there he was to find the Promised Land of Israel. Why "promised"? Because this was God's promise to us, once we had discovered and could claim the Ark of the Covenant that we had originally made with God.

When decoded through the sacred alphabet, the word "Israel" interprets through the scrolls as "through the intelligence of my Soul, I release and ascend my everlasting life" ("EL").

That is the story of how we began to birth our first integral genetic inheritance – this is where we are given the learned opportunity to understand the hidden strength of our mind, which also explains to us exactly what God is. The God "EL" was first recorded through the evolution of the myth.

A necessary digression here. Throughout my books, you will find equivalent stories as to how we evolved, and how we have had to learn to balance our thinking. Once again, I will remind you to please become used to the amount of quotation marks I apply in my books regarding my explanations of the codes of the Sacred Alphabet. More importantly, please become used to the continual references to the stories, where it may seem to you that I am repeating many of the same stories. Allow me to explain the reason for all of this. I am not repeating the same stories; each time you think I am repeating myself, you will find that I am advancing you into the next step of you attaining your freedom to release more of your DNA. Please read this sentence again, so that your ego can hear and understand why this is so. When you invisibly notice these quotations as you are reading, each word is automatically registered up into your unconscious mind. They become a reference library for your future, and then, every time you speak these words, you are harmonizing your central nervous system and mentally releasing the next step of your truth. While this is occurring, your intelligence climbs up another rung of its own ladder, which is your genetic inheritance of your individual DNA, and, through this, you evolve up into your inner dictionary, where you have an added interest that is given to you through your God self in order for you to initiate a desire to define the Divine.

As we come to rely on this education, we move forward to claim our inheritance; our inheritance is recorded in the Collective Consciousness, which is represented symbolically as the library in the city of Alexandria – and we now understand, through reading previous books in this volume, that this is explained syllable by syllable as the Mind of God. It was originally pronounced as "EL-Ex-AN-Dri-EA", which pertains to the first God, "EL", being introduced to the second God, "AN", and, through both of them harmonizing with one another through opening the heart to self, they became the third God, known to us mythically as "EA". Eventually, we began to notice, that "EA" is the crown of our head, which becomes our antenna, through the concordance of evolution. This inner school becomes our "Educational Faculty of Light", and, when we speak, we know that we are speaking through the confidence and truth that we have earned up to this point.

Please make sure that you drink plenty of water whilst reading my material, as, through your ego, the cells of your body are working overtime – as you begin to awaken into this higher hieroglyphical world – and you need to flush your thinking before it creates a disturbance in your energy. Accepting new information always dehydrates your body. Thank you for reading these preceding paragraphs of my digression.

Back we come to Moses, who was supposedly born into a poor family, and his mother placed him in a wicker basket on the river in order to save him from being killed by the soldiers of the Pharaoh. (Read the story in Exodus, chapter 2.) He floated down the river of life, and the daughter of Pharaoh found him in the bulrushes at the river's edge; metaphysically, the "daughter" represents the next thought of the Pharaoh's emotional mind. The baby's elder sister stood apart and watched this entire event taking place, and she stepped forward and said, "Shall I go and call to thee a nurse of the Hebrew women, that she may nurse the child for thee?" (Exodus 2:7) Pharaoh's daughter gave her permission, sending a maid with the girl to find the baby's mother, who then received wages to nurse him. And, as the child grew, the mother returned the child to Pharaoh's daughter. He became her son, and she named him Moses, as she said, "because I drew him out of the water." He was trained by the Temple Masters as an Architect, and his task was to build a great city for Pharaoh. (This also refers to the codes of the Master Mason, and we can see here how we began to connect to the beginnings of creating our Secret Societies.)

Now I will begin to explain the codes to deciphering the inner language. As he grew into his strength, Moses did not like the way that his grandfather, Pharaoh, handled the people who worked under him. Remember that the word "Pharaoh" is a later edition that has released through the inner dictionary from the word "King", which interprets as "key-ing"; the key opens the door, and which can also represent the "Chi" in God, announcing to us the Collective Energy that created God. Through the Arabic translations, this title was referred to as the "Sheik"; now this name interpreted as the "Shah" – or is it the same as the "Chi"; or is it how the same word is pronounced through a different personality or language being spoken at that time? And then we come to the last syllable of "Sheik" (i.e., "-ic"), and this syllable is explained to us as the "intelligence of creation"). The people of the land were devoid of their own emotional responsibility, their wisdom never had a chance to be free, and they lived under sufferance. The Pharaoh's ego was reigning supreme. Through his own dissatisfaction of understanding and accepting himself, he passed his own judgement out amongst his own constituency, as he had not yet earned his own responsibility for his thoughts; therefore, his right brain had not been acknowledged through his own intellect – which explains to us why he refused to acknowledge his own personalities, which, in turn, are interpreted metaphysically as his people. Now we can begin to understand how the penis had overstepped its own mark and begun to rule through its own supremacy.

The story continues, explaining to us that one day Moses caught one of the Egyptian guards abusing a Hebrew worker, and Moses got angry – angry enough for the stone that he threw at the guard to strike and kill the man. That was it – Moses had finally stood up for what he believed in! Further on in verse 13, we learn that the next day, when Moses returned to work, he was met by two Hebrews, one of whom said to him, "What you did was wrong! Why did you kill that man?" And then he went on to say, "Who made you a prince and a judge over us? Do you intend to kill me, as you did the Egyptian?"' And Moses said to him, "Surely you understand why I committed this act?" Again, we must understand the Metaphysical interpretation; the stone that Moses threw at the guard was a thought that released from his mind. We are now learning to balance the story through learning to understand that he did not kill the guard; he eradicated a thought that was trying to overpower another thought!

The two Hebrews who spoke with Moses the next day represent

our personalities that have evolved up intellectually and that are reigning supreme in their emotional understanding of self. When we look at the word "Hebrew" through the codes, we understand that these two are of the higher cast of our emotional intellect. Remember that "HE" is the heavenly energy, and "brew" is pertaining to "balance and release the eternal wisdom". These Hebrews – or personalities – were on the journey to begin to hear themselves, and they had been brought up to a higher level of their intellect; they were beginning to learn to take responsibility for their own actions. That is why they confronted Moses the next day regarding his having erased an extreme thought that had tried to take too much control of another personality.

When the Pharaoh heard this story of the guard who was struck down by Moses, he set out to slay him. "Moses fled from the face of Pharaoh and dwelt in the land of Midian; and he sat down by a well. Now the priest of Midian had seven daughters, and they came to the well and drew water and filled the troughs to water their father's flock." These seven daughters represent the seven emotional seals – or chakras – that we open up as we evolve up into the unconscious energy of the mind. So, please, allow me to awaken you into explaining more of the Metaphysical language.

Are you ready to add to your education – to hear, not just listen – as to how you will begin to understand much more astutely the Metaphysical interpretation of this story? Remember that the Pharaoh was the controlling influence of Egypt. Metaphysically, the word "Egypt" is known to us through the sacred codes as the "human body", and the Nile River represents our "spine". In the ancient language, the word "spine" was pronounced as "spinea". Could this wisdom have been understood, back then, as "the spin to 'EA'", or was it "the spine that represents 'EA'"? Pharaoh made all his people (which, again, symbolically refer to his own personalities) bow down and work for him. The reverence was created on his behalf was within himself, and this created his hierarchical mind. So, when he wanted to slay Moses – now let's get this one right; to slay means "to kill", and to kill means "to eradicate from the mind". Pharaoh wanted to eradicate Moses – or the thought/personality that Moses represented – from his mind. Through the interpretations that are explained in the Bible, when someone is killed, it means that a thought/personality was eradicated. In other words, the energy of that thought has been removed.

Do you think that the Bible was written to explain to us how we can kill another fellow human being? Please remember that this book was first written as a tablet for the person of higher mind in order to explain the "Divine language", which, again, is explaining the matter of physics, and we know that this is the language of the unconscious mind, which denotes as Metaphysics.

How about when God asks us to turn the other cheek! This denotes this way: When someone has struck at us, we are asked to "turn the other cheek"; in other words, do not strike back. Let us understand this hidden language first! And then we can judge what has already been specifically written in order for all of us to evolve into accepting our self.

So, Moses fled from the face of Pharaoh and dwelt in the land of "Mid-i-an", as it is written in the Bible. Why the "face"? The nerves which are collected in our face represent every organ in our body; these organs are our Inner Universes complying with our own justice, which is reflected back to us – that is, when we look into a mirror, we see our own reflection. Now let's take a look at the syllables. Mid means "middle"; i means "intelligence"; an is the "centre of the Soul" and the "home of our educational mind" (connecting to the name of the second God, "AN"). The verse does not state "Pharaoh"; therefore, in this story, he is not referred to as a separate identity. So now we are noticing that the explanation, through the matter of physics or the Metaphysical equation, is that the whole story of Moses is an emotional birthright – that is, an explanation of a personality that is part of Pharaoh's emotional mind. This is expressed through the language of the right hemisphere of the brain, and, of course, we refer to this hemisphere as our subconscious mind. All this information will become an estimated earning for Pharaoh, as well as an educational lesson for his grandson. Remember that it was Pharaoh's daughter (emotional mind) who claimed Moses as her son; and, thus, he grew up in the land of Egypt.

Are you awakening to this inner sound? Please read slowly, and have the patience to go over the text, again and again, until you begin to "hear" my words. Don't just listen – listening to someone only registers in the left ear, which supports the left brain. That means your ego is looking at! Hearing comes through the right ear, and this registers with the right brain. Once you hear these words, they will equate mathematically and release up into your unconscious aspect of self. This intelligence will become your wisdom, and it will remain on standby – that is, available to you forevermore. Now you will understand that you are learning to look through, not at! Remember that our intelligence is an acquired position that we reach, through our mind being harmonized, as both the left and right hemispheres of our brain come together and work as one. This is the hierarchical mind collecting your endowment.

The many doctors and medical students who come to see me are adding this information to their own training, especially as to how they can understand and refer to many of the dis-eases that we are so busily creating. It explains to them the reasoning behind the dis-ease, and it opens up the possibilities to rearrange the initial program of why each dis-ease presented itself to the body through the first initiation; I do hope that this is the introduction into experiencing the growth of futuristic medicine. Please remember; I am introducing you to the language of the unconscious recognition of self; this is the language of the Soul; the sole – or Soul – reason why we are here is to earn the experience of consciousness in order to carry forward the consequences of our thinking to create the energetic future of the planet! This allows a totally different perspective for you to view, as it is the opposite of what you have learned throughout your life while existing in the third-dimensional reality. The unconscious mind is your mirror reflecting back to you. Now you can understand when I say, "Reverse your questions, and you will receive the correct answer." This is how our inner vision begins to transfer the inner language back to us; the more we depend on it, the more it broadens – and, through multiplication, it extols our own virtue. Before you step up into this higher realm of intellect it is known to you as the "language of your dreams".

Back to the story. When Moses arrived in the land of Midian, he sat down by a well. As we open up into the inner language, we find that a well is a symbol of one of the first examples of the unconscious mind; it explains the reflection of life, and then it releases this vision down to you. The well, a hole in the ground, was first created as a place to hold water. Thus, we created the well, leaning over it with a long rope connected to a bucket, and then we drew the water up and out. Through time, we created a spindle to work on our behalf, which took away the heaviness of drawing up the water; this made life much easier. The water is used as an example through the ancient myths; symbolically, it represents the deep, dark section of our consciousness. It is hidden under the ground, which is where we are relying on our past to fulfil us. This is why most of the tales that came from long ago usually tell us about someone in a ship crossing the ocean, such as in the Greek epic poems of Homer, the Odyssey and the Iliad (we are aware of Odysseus visit to the Cyclops), among many others.

Now let us explain the "Priest of Midian", who, along with his seven daughters, drew water from the well to water their flock. We go on to read that the "shepherds came and drove them away: but Moses stood up and helped them to water their flock". The daughters took Moses back to their father and explained that he had helped them water the flock, and the father was grateful and gave Moses one of his daughters, who went by the name of Zipporah, for a wife. Every sentence we read is explaining the codes of how Moses learned to balance his mind. So Moses lived with his new family and birthed his first son, who was named Gershom, and reared the priest's flock.

I am not going to explain each chapter, as it will take many pages for me to interpret all of it; however, we now have an explanation of what Moses represents, metaphysically, in the Old Testament. The Bible goes on to explain how God was pleased with Moses, and an angel appeared in the burning bush – which represents the resurrection of the self – and explained to Moses that he had to return to Egypt to bring the children of Israel out of Egypt and into the land flowing with milk and honey.

The decision was made to take the people who had befriended him during his childhood to the Promised Land, and Pharaoh agreed. So Moses gathered the Hebrews together, and off they went across the Red Sea to the other side. The Red – or the Sea of Reeds – represents the ending of one life to begin another. Or, through Metaphysics, it is interpreted as the ending of one thought, once it has been fully expressed, in order to begin again through the next thought.

The journey supposedly took forty years to accomplish; once again, we are explaining the codes. The number forty (40) interprets as the "Temple of the Soul". Now this journey, when it is explained to you through the mathematics of Metaphysics, was for Moses to reach his "Temple House" or "Home". It is explaining to you that Moses began his inner journey, travelling up through his DNA in order to discover himself through releasing his inner intelligence.

That is where the troubles began, and it is where they still are to this very day, thousands of years later. Nobody understood the hidden language, so how could they understand the mathematical codes of the mind? This is the story of the evolution of humanity's DNA! Again, there is only one story. We are still waking up to a parable told many light years ago. Moses is symbolically representing the "Penis", taking his people – or his "Semen", which symbolically represents his next thought – to the Promised Land. In other words, his semen or seed had to be saved. Thus, through our innocence of not understanding what God portended for us, we have been had! This is the beginning of the first God, "EL", and it is a story written long, long ago– and remember that "EL" and represents our "Everlasting Life".

***

The story continues to explain itself in the Gospel of Matthew, which is the first book of the New Testament. There was a King at that time whose name was Herod – or "He-Rod". He wanted to kill all the male children in order to keep his power for himself. When he was told that a new Messiah had been born in Bethlehem, it did not sit well with him, as he knew that a new Messiah would usurp him from his own position. He did

14

not wish to have to surrender to this next positive thought, so he called his wise men and sent them out to search for the newborn child. He said to them, "When you have found him, send me word so that I may come and worship him also." The wise men travelled to meet the new Messiah, whose name was Jesus ("He-Zeus"), and they gave him gifts of "gold, frankincense, and myrrh".

They never returned to report back to Herod; they left for a new land instead. The new Messiah's father, who was known as Joseph, had a vision from an angel, who told him to leave Bethlehem and go into Egypt, as the old King Herod wanted to kill his son. So Joseph, along with his wife (Mary), fled to safety with the child. The story then goes on to explain how Herod then sent out his army to kill every boy-child in the land. Herod was satisfied with himself, and so did not want to change his stature; through the matter of physics – or Metaphysics – his rigid thinking would not allow his next positive thought to change his current identity.

Now you can see where the story of Moses of the Old Testament begins, and where it ends in the New Testament with Jesus. Moses is explaining to us how we can understand ourselves, and Jesus is the result or the action. This is the "Testes" or the "Testicle"; the Testament of the Oracle that is embedded in our cells.

Your Notes:

CHAPTER THREE

The "G(OD) Spot"

The stories in the books of Mathew, Mark, Luke, and John all differ, through the intellectual interpretation of the arcing of each of their minds; in other words, the authors write through their individual Metaphysical interpretation of their own emotional stability. Thus we see that it is the same story as to how Jesus learned to understand the relationship of gathering himself together and arcing his way up to facing his own responsibilities; however, we also see that each author explains that story through different emotions. Maybe now you can understand why my words are repeated through different emotions.

In the innocence of discovering our own inner freedom of self, the lower ancient half of our bodies starts to awaken, and we begin the journey to understand ourselves. We learn to ignite our sexuality, as this promotes our primal urge to spring to our own attention – these feelings instigate our personalities to become more aware, which helps us to characterize our thinking. These feelings come from the second evolutionary level of our brain awakening, and the way in which they transfer the responsibility of our intellect up into the third brain – which, as we know, is the unconscious mind.

When we commit to the sexual act, that act clears the guardians of the old channels of our consciousness; it reduces our stubbornness, which allows us to birth through and beyond our primordial mind of the moment. Our emotional mind comes alive, where we learn to release our feelings, and this can only happen when we learn to open our heart to our self! It is like an inner rain that flushes through the body and cleanses the cells. The act of sex is enhancing the lesser Gods within. Those lesser Gods explode into their light – or intellect – where they have been given the right to harmonize and balance up into the Collective Mind of self. Einstein's "Theories of Relativity" rebound again!

We step onto the next level of our pathway when we are

dissatisfied with ourselves and out of balance with our lives. We feel that there is nothing happening, or that we are just not good enough, and so we begin the next part of our journey by questioning ourselves as to how we can open up these layers of confinement through rearranging these levels of our intellect.

Sexual dissatisfaction gives us the courage to turn our attention back inside ourselves and revisit the fear that is hanging in suspension, and then we begin to collate the promises that we would like to accomplish and return back into ourselves.

We become more aware of how the orgasm and ejaculation release, cleansing every cell in our body, through the strength that collects through our feelings regarding our self! The vibrations of the orgasm – or the Godness – then sends that energy up through the body to the crown of the head, and this act completely enhances and rebalances the ego of self. The word "orgasm" means "through the Oracle releasing God, we ascend up into the Soul's measurement". To achieve that orgasm, your heart has the opportunity to open up to collect the feelings that then create the feeling of total enlightenment.

The Apostle Peter (in the Bible) and the God P'tah (from the principles of Egypt) are connected to the heart, as they both represent the dove, which, in Shamanism, empowers the totem to polarize and ground the energetic fields of the body. It is pure God essence, which is created through all the lesser Gods earning the intellectual right to move up and meld into becoming one God. It is when we are at that orgasmic point that our cells can reverberate to gather their own light and release the fear of the moment. Throughout the orgasm and ejaculation, we give ourselves the opportunity to lift ourselves up into the higher realms of our own expectations, and that essence of God is what we are capable of achieving on our Quest of Life.

It is when the fear that we have within us becomes infatuated with its own personality of self that we relate to what we call the "infidel" in the Bible. That infidel is our own ego, vying for its own superior control over the rest of the body. The sexual energy becomes our overtone, and it must be heard; thus, we must learn to co-exist with all our personalities in order to accomplish and release the freedom of self. Through our intelligence, our personalities are numerous; thus, when we become afraid of our own virtue, the infidel – or the ego – steps forward to gain control over all.

As this experience vibrates up through the meridian lines in our body, we begin to realize that it is to the detriment of our own freedom that we subside back into yearning for the primal odour of our own excuses. If only we could allow and trust the embodiment of self to achieve this ultimate state of wisdom for us!

An Orgasm is a climactic impulse that aligns inside the vagina, reaching up, out, and through to the clitoris. That energy, through the blessing that we return to ourselves during intercourse, becomes a form of cognitional therapy, and it is this inheritance that stimulates and creates the strength within, not the blessing that you are trying to give to your partner.

If the energy is harmonized through one another, then the unconscious mind can collectively liberate both of you at the same time. That is one of the miracles, or religious experiences, that we can receive when we open our heart to the vibrations of what we are feeling through love. Nicely said, don't you think? (The explanation that I have been given to describe this is that "we aqueate our senses"; no, aqueate is not in the dictionary, so let us look at the make-up of the word to interpret that it means we are "able to liberate ourselves from the inner waters of our own consciousness.") The journey of enlightenment is to move the energy found in the clitoris or penis up to the third eye – or the pineal gland – both of which are equal to the unconscious mind in their relationship through one another.

Enlightenment is the centred mind – it is the silent mind of the Guru, the Avatar, and the Shaman – and this area is more popularly referred to as the "Eye of God". It is best explained, symbolically, through myth as the unicorn. Throughout the parables, it is our own Spiritual strength – which is the horse in the Shamanic language – bringing the sexual energy up into the third eye ("Eye of God"). The spiralled horn of the unicorn symbolically represents the power that we attain through releasing our own intelligence and stepping up into the Collective; this purifies the DNA embedded in our bones. Could this also relate to what I have written a few pages back regarding the word "Spinea"?

Again, it is also an explanation of the Egyptian word "Bja", which has been interpreted as "the iron in our bones". This is the "metal energy" that is spoken of through the Chinese language. It is the collection of our inner strength. Christianity refers to it as the "devil"; but, if we reverse that word, we will see that it becomes the word "lived", which is in reference to our past, and which becomes our bank of memories. The species of animal that produce horns have reached their own completion when they birth those horns – that is, through the compatibility of the unconscious mind, they are already living collectively.

This energy is brought up through to the pituitary gland, and, through the stimulation, our feelings become the collected strength; this is then carried up into our pineal gland, and, from there, it erupts out into the brain, which begins to clear and change the Alchemy that has collected but has not been used to its own fulfilment throughout the eclectic pathways. The reasoning behind this is that we are thinking the same thought over again, but we are not doing anything positive with these thoughts. This energy builds up in our primal sexual behaviour, where we are urged to commit back into the sexual act again to regain that brief moment of enlightenment which enhances these pathways of our intellect. When we have balanced the mind, we find a completion that encompasses our thoughts, and we become an enlightened being. And, until we learn to stop running away from the responsibility of what we are thinking – but not doing – we will find that we have jammed up the works once again.

Just as the volcano erupts from the centre of the earth to clear its own pressure – which has collected through its energy mounting up into becoming a stressful situation that is not being realized – we, too, achieve the same effect when the orgasm or ejaculation explodes throughout the cells of our body.

I have learned that women build up to release the orgasm in five areas, not just one. Men have only two areas. Inside the vagina, these five areas are recognized through the echo of the lymphatic system, which, in turn, forwards this into the glands. Our sexual energy is then collected to create a sequence of vibrations, which work their way up to accumulate into what we refer to as the "G(OD) Spot".

During the education of our first-dimensional mind, this area is known as our "gravity centre"; it is where our mathematics equate and release the energy up into these upper sections of glandular inheritance, as they busily vibrate through the energetic pathways where our neurons are surged through waves of expectation, opening up to connect and release into the cellular mind. The more we relax into this awakening, the more those five vortexes of energy are collectively unleashed and opened. It is the vibration that swells the mucous membranes, which unite with one another to create the atomic explosions inside the body. It is the woman who is receiving, while the man is releasing.

Our cells cluster and release their mucus inheritance. The sexual flow of energy is carried up into the area of the pituitary gland, which is mathematically balancing and harmonizing this pure energy, so that the vibrations are swathed back down to release the juices through the vagina. As it is with the sexual yearning, so, too, is it with us as we learn to accept the sacred knowledge of our body. What is stimulated through the lower half of the body must be reimbursed to the upper half, which then corrects the Alchemy of the brain. We are permanently balancing the energy to create the symbol of infinity, which is creating the harmonic balance of our Soul's knowledge.

We use exactly the same energy when we are releasing our intellect up into our crown chakra, where we can touch our forehead with the tips of our fingers, and, through the mathematics of the Alchemy reaching their own zenith, we are able to create an orgasm. It is called the path of ecstasy, and is a great way to fly!

Sex, at the peak of its perfection, is the orgasmic cloud of the heavenly kingdoms of your God within anointing itself through you. That is the totality of your ego entering into the light of self in order for you to receive your enlightenment.

The cervix has the same power as a black hole in the Universe, and women have the gift of creating and releasing that power. My teachers taught me that, as a woman reaches the peak of orgasm, it is unconsciously registered in the minds of every other woman on the planet. Just as the whale, as it swims in the ocean, is able to communicate with every other whale. When my teachers told me that, I found it hard to believe or accept, and I replied, "Goodness, isn't anything secret or sacred?" The answer from my teachers was, "No, not to the unconscious mind. These subtle vibrations are light beams of intellect that reflect out to same mind, and this stimulation helps to lift and cleanse the blocked emotions in those of us who are replacing the sexual act with another excuse."

Sex cleanses every cell in your body; it vibrates every nerve that is out of alignment, and it brings the body back up into being able to look into its own perfection.

Some of us seem to have a fear of getting to know ourselves. We are afraid to bring our sexual thinking up into our Spiritual essence, and so we keep on allowing others to manipulate us. Learn to feel good about yourself. Get to know your body telepathically, and then ask yourself some questions. Your sex is your own ego searching for its own wisdom and belief, so turn your ego on!

Your Notes:

CHAPTER FOUR

The Orgasmic Cloud

Women speak to me regarding their childhood sexual abuse, after they have become devastated emotionally through locking that thought inside. I like to explain to them why their personalities had to be kept hidden for so long. When we keep them hidden, we refrain from taking part in the womanly enterprise, and so we remain the child. The woman – the symbolic Sekhmet and Hathor energy, as explained through the Egyptian principles – cannot bring through her own development. There are millions of unhappy women out there who have still not found their glory within. They permanently live a lie to themselves, and this is where their fear overrides their inner satisfaction.

Sekhmet is that wanton woman, the Siren; she is the Goddess of ego and pride, the Lion woman. In the Egyptian hieroglyphs, Sekhmet is the Goddess of the Upper Universe, also known as the Goddess of Justice. The reigning garment that she symbolically wears was created through the 10,000 eyes that come from the tail of the peacock. She is a powerful woman who knows how to strut her stuff; she is the deity of sex. Likewise, her opposite emotional partner, through the myths, is Hathor the Cow. The cow represents our inner contentment, so her partner is receiving and balancing the contentment that she gives back to herself.

Mary Magdalene is another familiar thought form; she is the woman inside you who wants to feel and be touched. She is also a yearning. The word "Magdalene" means the "master ascending through God's Divine ascension, living her energy through nourishing herself emotionally." In other words, she is the emotion of giving and receiving the sexual flow. She is the first teacher of imploding the light within! Do not leave her locked inside; allow her to release her energy. Let your thinking expand into your consciousness in order for your freedom to accomplish its own achievements.

It is just a matter of changing your thinking; it is now time for you to get over the insecurities that you are hiding behind and release the freedom that has collected from this inner education of accepting yourself. When you see your partner again, push your light right through that house and cover him with it – then smile and strut your stuff!

The clitoris speaks to us through great wisdom. First, you must free yourself in order to accomplish it, and then you must understand how to feel at ease in yourself in order to release it. It speaks to us through the crown it has created as a result of these five areas of expediency surging forward. How can a man know what you want if the symbol is not vibrated out, into, and through your layers? What you think, so you attract – so brighten up your thinking. Do you want that guy to want to share some of his time with you? If so, make sure your thinking is ahead of you, so that he can trip over it!

A wonderful Merlin energy awakens within us on this journey of life, and it allows us to look at the world without judgement; we begin to see what our truth really is – the dances that we co-create behind the veils of how we interpret what we think. The word "Merlin" – or, more correctly, as it was collected through the words "Mer-EL-AN", once it was decoded – means that the Meer – or ocean of consciousness – of the God "EL" opens up through intellectually nurturing the home of self, which is the mythical home of the God "AN". As we have intellectually progressed through time and accepted the codes, we then changed the pronunciation of the letter a to i. All this means that the "oceans of consciousness" bring you everlasting life when you come home to the inn to rest.

In the ancient language, the word "inn" was originally pronounced as "Airn"; hence, the word "bairn", meaning "young child" – or, allowing the self to birth, to be born again. Throughout history the sacred coding is automatically registered in our mind and symbolically envisaged as an old man (i.e., Merlin), so that symbol represents the Collective Power that we have encoded within ourselves. This wonderful Merlin energy teaches us how to produce the magic of our own "royal behaviour" – that is, how we are able to achieve our own satisfaction through the feeling of self-love eternally creating and balancing the self. It works with us, not against us! Look at the "Aum" symbol that so many of us proudly wear around our neck these days. The word "Aum", when decoded, means "ascending, understanding, and mastering". This symbol is an introduction into balancing the Collective Mind of God (throughout other languages this symbol is represented as "OM").

The Mind of God, through the codes, is the balance of "EL", the everlasting life, which is the introduction into the lungs of consciousness up through the sexual doorway, which travels up into the "Airn", which is now called "AN". Remember that Airn means ascending through intelligence through releasing and nourishing, and it is the home of the second symbolic recognition of God. It then travels up through the awakening of the heart to traverse up into the crown, which is the home of "EA".

Those three mythical centres – "EL-AN-EA" – create the Oracle of the mind. There are still a few of the old languages spoken on the planet, and those who pronounce their words through these ancient kingdoms will stay here on the planet until their language is recognized through the next generation of intellect. Once their language has been understood correctly, they will notice that they have the opportunity to expand their own DNA, which will change the history lessons for the next generation of their tribe.

The same symbol in the Asian vibration is Yin/Yang, which is correctly pronounced as "Airn/Eang" through the Asian language. Once again, we symbolically refer to the sexual and spiritual thinking perfectly balancing as one, which is explained through the Asian principles as a pronounced harmonic channel through which they communicate to the creator. It is the educated mind, which is free of its sexual manipulation, and so is able to create and allow its new language to be delivered unto them.

Now you can begin to see how every language on the planet is sonically connected through the atmospheric inheritance of the Collective Mind. All of which is the gift we are given through the art of telepathic communication.

Many Asian cultures consider sex an excusable religion, where their primal mind has the opportunity to become educated through empowering the thought of the moment. As we learn to heighten our intelligence, we use our sexual energy to open up, and, with this internal empowerment, we are able to release our inner wisdom. Your clitoris and penis – both of which are the beginning of, and the first important doorway to, your Spiritual pathway – create the Collective Energy that travels straight up to the solar plexus. This energy then nestles in the Soul area of the God "AN", and, through educating the self, it gathers in momentum and is carried forward, up, into, and through the heart.

We cannot see these energy lines (meridians) until we begin this next quest of intellectual knowledge. These meridians are subtle vibrations that collect and gather in the big toe, and the feelings travel up through to the inner thighs, through to the vagina and penis, and then traverse up into the constellation of the Soul; the heart begins its subtle vibrations, and our feelings are swept up into the pituitary gland, where they are collected, weighed, and measured through the mathematical stimulation – and then they have the opportunity to release into the pineal gland. The overflow of this stimulated energy is then swilled around throughout the neurons of the brain, which autonomically changes the Alchemy of the mind, and we learn how to reside in peace. These meridians are what we refer to as the "light of the angelic resonance", which can very quickly become stigmatized – or trapped – through your fear of you not knowing how to release your inner wisdom. And this can very quickly become a social disgrace through the inner collection of the uninitiated adolescent – or your innocent mind. Why hide from yourself?

Just above the heart is the thymus gland, and, when this gland is connected through the sacred codes, the word "thymus" means: "thy must be true to thyself". We may be able to fake an orgasm on an outer level to our partner, but we cannot fake it inside ourselves. If you cannot bring the orgasmic cloud created on your behalf up through the heart area – where it is recognized for what is happening in your body, and from where it is then carried through to the thymus gland – the energy cannot come up into the crown. This means that the Alchemy does not switch on inside the brain, and the area that is then in control of our senses is the pituitary gland. Remember the previous story: If you do not get your thoughts right, all is tipped back into the left hemisphere of your brain, where you have to live the experience over again until you do get it right! Why pass on your fears to your daughter?

The thymus gland has to receive the vibrations from the orgasmic cloud, and, if it doesn't, it refuses to allow the healing to take place – and the energy from the orgasm just swims around inside your body, going straight back to where it came from. Only half the body becomes satisfied, so it creates a lack of sexual satisfaction. We are then on the way to creating endometriosis in women, and prostate problems in men (through the swelling of the prostate gland) – both of which are the precursor to diabetes. (One in five of us are now accepting this dis-ease of diabetes, which is continually advancing.

Your Notes:

CHAPTER FIVE

Mary Magdalene

We read stories in the Bible regarding two women with the same name: Mary. Jesus' mother is Mary, and the other Mary is Mary Magdalene (from whom were cast the seven devils). The mother Mary represents the right brain, and Mary Magdalene represents the Sekhmet (ego and pride) of the left brain.

Mary Magdalene had to earn her own victory of educated intelligence; this is the explanation written in the Bible of the casting out of the seven devils, which metaphorically relate to the seven seals, through her releasing and cleansing her own attitude towards self. Once she has conformed to her own state of grace, of course, she then becomes an Apostle, as no negative memory remains on which she needs to rely! (This happens to each of us as we conform to our own state of grace.) The "magda" is the emotional magician, the woman who lives in the earthly kingdoms and nourishes herself on her sexuality. She was known as a whore – and remember that whores were used in the ancient writings to represent those emotional thoughts, which were abused through the thoughts of the ego searching for more excuses for itself! And, as we know today, when we mention the word "whore" in communicating with others, we find it is used as a resting place for the ego, through its judgemental nature, to conform to its own grace!

Mary Magdalene's story – which receives only a cursory description in the Bible – has been reinvented endlessly down through the ages, as we have still not understood the Metaphysical language that was explained to us in the original telling. She is briefly mentioned as the one who went to the tomb three days after Jesus supposedly died; and this is where and when she received her vision – she saw Jesus alive again! A vision is something we view from within. It is a knowing that we receive from our Higher Self! Jesus was supposedly buried in the tomb in the garden of Joseph of Arimathea. So I will explain this legend as well.

Through the Arabic language, Joseph is denoted as "Youseph". The word "Youseph" interprets as "yourself"! Arimathea explains the "aromatics we produce and receive from the heavenly 'EA". Thus, through the Metaphysical interpretation, Jesus had died, and his "arithmetics" had returned him to his heavenly home. The two Marys represent the "matriarch" and the "wanton Goddess", both of whom dwell within all women. The mother Mary sometimes dampens man's enthusiasm because she lacks ardour, and yet, she is there to comfort men when they are in doubt regarding their own confinement. The word "mother" is also the word "martyr" – that is, the one who is in sacrifice to herself through constantly giving to others. A man does not want to make love to his mother, but he would not mind getting to know Mary Magdalene every once in a while.

Mary Magdalene, again, is the magician, who, through her desires, is earning her Divine ascension; she is also able to define the Divine in the vagina. That explanation is also explained in the hieroglyphs on the back walls of the Temple of Hathor in the ancient city of Danderra, Egypt – or "Tanterra" ("tantra"), as it is known throughout the Indian-Buddhist religions. It is explaining to us the codes to the temple of sexuality. Mary Magdalene represents the emotion "Desire", and the mother Mary represents the emotion "Divine".

It has taken more than 1,500 years to try to understand the stories explained to us in the Bible, and that is why it is still the most popular book on the planet. The Bible, along with the hieroglyphs on the walls of the temples in Egypt, reveals the hidden codes. It is all the same story, and that story can only be revealed through us entering up into the next phase of the hidden intelligence.

***

Our minds have become much more knowledgeable and scientific in this age, and through our being able to understand that all those stories are about the evolution of the human being, we are bringing religion and science together. As our intelligence aligns with the past, we are finding that more of the past is opening up in order to reveal itself. The veils are lifting to release these restrictions, which, through our innocence, we have kept bound. They are stories about you opening up your glandular systems to allow you to become your light. Light is intelligence; and, when you use your Soul energy along with intelligence, the combination becomes an emotional inheritance that will be passed on to your next generation.

Emotions are something that you have the ability to create through the feelings that release when you are living an experience. Before the heart can be opened, it must be able to attach itself to the respect that you have for your self. Emotions collect mathematically in order for you to be able to release these feelings. Feelings create a sensuous vibration that frees the heart of the restrictions that you, for your own security, have placed around you. So, the more of you that understand these passages, the fewer heart attacks that the rest of the population will create.

When you go out to search for a relationship, know that the other person has his/her own difficulties to deal with as well. Know also that you are not responsible for his/her difficulties, nor should you interfere with that person's life. There should be a sense of freedom to create this relationship, in which both of you can find and reach your own stability.

When you enter into a relationship, and the changes begin, remember to always give thanks to yourself in order for that relationship to bring both of you together. When you give yourself to your partner, the energy returns back to you, through the cognition of the unconscious mind. If you want a relationship to last, please take the time to find someone who is equivalent to your own level. The greatest word I use with clients who have come for advice regarding their relationship is "respect". This word has far-reaching consequences, as it comes to us in two syllables: re- is "to return", and -spect is "to look through", not at. When we look "at", remember that we are creating another excuse to judge; by looking "through", we release, in ourselves, the truth of that person.

When you attract a person into your life, understand what energetic responses you were searching for at the time that you called him/her into your life; as you sow, so shall you reap, and, as you think, so shall it become. Did you know that you have had a prior right to meet every person you have ever met in your life? That is the Collective Consciousness releasing and enhancing your disabilities through where you are not understanding your Divine self. We are "Tribal Emporia" holding ourselves in abeyance as to what is expected of us.

Somewhere, enveloped in your DNA, is a reference – or code of conductivity – that will enable you to home in on the same tribal gatherings of mind as your own. It collects itself over the generations, and it only works through the unconscious mind. Thus, your ancestors have already contacted everyone that you meet throughout your life – long before you even entered into the scene – which has already measured itself with the Collective, in order for you to meet their next generations in this lifetime. Energy attracts attention.

Finding someone on the same level of emotional intelligence as you are is a difficult experience, through you being automatically drawn to the person, sensing what you do not want to acknowledge or see in your self – and this experience is what you need to be brought to your attention, in that moment. We become smitten with one another. This word "smitten" needs explaining. Through the Old English language, and up until the thirteenth century, it meant "to soil or stain oneself'. In today's thinking, it means "to be struck or hit hard". So, when we become smitten, it means that we are being abruptly pulled out of own safety and security.

Your Notes:

CHAPTER SIX

Marriage

The term "marriage" means "the joining of two links"; my sons taught me this word when they were learning to weld. They said, "To make a strong chain, the links must always be welded equally; otherwise, when one link becomes weak, the join will break."

To get those two links to meld together, one needs a bright light. The same as the weld! We refer to that light as a collection of supersonic vibrations being stimulated into its own power; we have named it "Love" – that is, where you are "living the Oracle of your life", and that is the secret to a successful marriage! If you are free enough within your self to each be able to love your partner unconditionally, then it is a perfect match, through both of you having served your self first, in order to be able to join with one another equally.

Marriage is not God-made; it is man's way of equalizing a shared responsibility through, and with, God's eyes. A marriage is about the nourishing and nurturing of one another.

Marriages are ending more now than at any other time, as a result of women releasing their intellectual abilities through learning to regale their thinking to support their inner strength. A failed marriage is never a mistake. The word "failed" creates guilt, and you are guilty of nothing. You or your partner had an awakening, where one of you outgrew the other; as a result, instead of an experience that you have earned, the marriage becomes a burden.

Let me tell you a story about how relationships can fail. A male and female are walking down the street, and they meet. The first thing one does is to notice the eyes of the other, which is where we are looking at one another through the windows of the Soul. Try to remember to always look at each other right eye to right eye, as the right eye is the window to the Soul, as this energy stems from the right hemisphere of the brain, which connects to our inner thoughts, which allows you to emotionally view each other's truth.

Don't bother with the left eye; that is the eye of the ego, and, very quickly, you will begin to realize that this person is reflecting back to you what you are searching for within yourself.

Back to that couple. They travel down the road, playing happily together, until they notice that a pause begins to create itself and extend in the relationship. She hears something he has said, which does not register with her own thoughts, and she thinks, "I did not realize he thought like that. I will have to sit with that remark for a while." And the pause becomes immiscible throughout their contact with one another. He also walks along and hears something she says, which does not register with his thoughts, and he thinks, "Where the hell did that remark come from? I did not know she thought like that!"

From that point, they begin to walk away from each other, through the one's ego flaring up to contend with the other, which strangles each other's emotions. But, somewhere deep inside, through viewing each other through the right eye, they each know that they have a Soul connection with the other, and so they try to overview their discrepancies and come back together again. This is where the sexual contact vies for supremacy, and we have overlapped the moment. The moment continues until one or the other, through understanding themselves in a clearer light, accepts their thoughts and then feels free to move on.

You do not have the right to judge anyone else; the word "judgement" is embedded in the first God's dictionary, where you release the word when you create an excuse for yourself! Through your intellectual light, you should never interfere with another Soul's journey. Share your intelligence with each other, but do not leach each other out. By sharing your intelligence with each other, you are mastering the relationship, and your marriage will always direct you down another pathway to gain a new experience. When the sharing stops, the decline of that relationship begins to seat itself.

When I had become a teenager, my grandmother explained to me that, when an argument between us was about to announce itself, we should hold hands with one another. We were not to use our left hands, only our right; and we would find, by holding each other's right hand, that the argument was over before it began. Both egos cannot compete with this unconscious recognition of telepathic enhancement.

In my seminars, I explain to my students about the power of love that we each have the opportunity to give to our self. I teach them how to empower this emotion that we have named "Love", which is where we are given the opportunity to eternally master the light of self.

Each person who comes into your life in a relationship is meant to be there, as there are lessons in your life that you still have to learn. The Universal Law has invited them into your life in order for you to learn how to become balanced and harmonized. You are being pulled out of your old world of thought in order to reveal and release the next step of your own creation.

Through accepting your partner, you are receiving the parts of yourself that are still lacking, which is why the ego is relying on a relationship to convert itself! Through the two of you being drawn together in a partnership, you create a new temple of light for both of you.

Your Notes:

CHAPTER SEVEN

Children

The children that are conceived within a relationship coincide with the emotions that you have attained up to that moment; they become a reflection of you and your partner. Through the inner weakness that you have surrendered your thoughts to, you are programming to bring your children through to face the responsibilities that you were too afraid to see. Through the temperament of the unconscious mind, which is our Soul, we acquiesce to inherit from the parent. Remember that the childish attitude births the child. Mother's fear subsides once the baby is born, as she has someone totally dependent on her to occupy her mind, and so she grows up and collects that added responsibility to rear the child. Father is happy, as he has the family lineage continually moving into his future.

You manifest the Soul of your child through your thinking. When we "collapse" and "fall" pregnant, that embryo must receive its Soul energy, and that Soul energy is delivered to us through the Collective Consciousness. The Universal Law is mirroring back to us the answer to our thoughts. Do you understand that sentence? This is the genetic inheritance that we receive from God. That Soul has, in its program, the embedded inheritance to live out both the negative and positive aspects of the parents' behaviour.

You, as your parents' children, have chosen to live your parents' lives; you have the responsibility of clearing the results of their past actions through advancing your own. You have chosen to live their fears, and, along the way, to release their burdens. All of which becomes the collected strength of humanity – to train and advance the ego into supplementing to the wholeness of self through the left hemisphere of the brain, "not" through the emotional right brain. Now you will feel more applicable, in regard to understanding your parents' thinking and learning from the information, as to why you feel tempted to design your own signature.

Before we go on, please realize that we have never made a

mistake; we have gained a tremendous amount of experience as to understanding the hidden truth in this Universal Law of Self.

Let me explain that paragraph further. In all relationships, one must release to the other; we are not all on the same level of emotional intelligence. We do not understand each other's Law of Self, although we do acknowledge and earn the Spiritual togetherness that makes a relationship feel complete. We begin that process by creating a séance of our thoughts, in the hope of equalizing both minds.

We begin to fall in love as the heart and mind become entwined, and, in the beginning stages of the relationship, we release and send our energy to the other person. This is accomplished through how often we think about them. While we are thinking of them, we begin to interrupt their thoughts, so that they, in return, begin to think of us. The man's ego begins to step up as he commits himself to the relationship: "I am beginning to feel a responsibility in this relationship; therefore, I have a commitment to look after this woman." After they marry and settle down together, he knows that he has her safely enveloped within him, and that knowledge gives him his peace of mind and self-satisfaction.

Many women who stay at home after marriage very quickly become bored through their idleness, because they do not have enough to do to keep their minds occupied. I have heard that story a thousand-plus times. They feel penned in; their emotions choke them down, and they begin to create stress in their body.

Whilst she allows her man to control her, the wife is considered to be a "good girl". When she realizes that she cannot comply with her own thinking, her emotions begin to become overloaded, choking her, and that "good girl" then sacrifices herself to have a child. Two years later, she has another child – all through her not feeling satisfied with her own answers. If the relationship of self is still not working out, another pregnancy occurs, and another – until she realizes and understands her emotional dilemma's much better. So, until we have intellectually moved forward, God or these wonderful laws of the universe, which decodes as –the Greatness of the Oracle of the Divine-, will keep on directing our mathematical flow of life.

Pregnancy is you hanging onto one thought for too long before birthing – or ascending – into your next thought. You will not let your old thinking go; you have become too settled and comfortable with your thinking, to the point where you do not have the confidence to allow the next positive thought to begin. Alternatively, if you are in a relationship where both of you feel the contentment of being with one another, through creating your own happiness, then you and your partner are free to love and become one. It is when you step out of alignment with yourself, looking for excuses for the momentary thoughts that need repairing, that the pregnancy occurs. Through the next level of intelligence releasing itself, we find that it is all about you experiencing your own mind and releasing your freedom within.

I was shocked to learn, during my education, that I had opened the doorway and allowed myself to become pregnant three months before each of my pregnancies occurred. I then had to face up to and learn how my thoughts, at that time, gave each of my children their ego and emotions. Through mirroring my own thinking to them, I had manifested their emotional ups and downs.

At that stage of my life, through my acceptance of each of my pregnancies, I felt happy, and so I birthed strong children. At that time, I felt that I was doing the right thing. But, when things were difficult in the relationship and I was feeling unhappy regarding the pregnancy, I birthed children that had difficulty swallowing and digesting their own emotions. I now know the consequences that they must abide by. Those are another set of values that we add to our lessons in life, and, when we understand and accept our own discernment, we learn to birth the right in the self to move on! Our children then spend the rest of their lives mirroring back to us the discrepancies that we created through our innocence of learning to understand ourselves!

Through your dissatisfaction in trying to repair the damages that you are thinking and creating, your saliva vibrates at a faster rate. That vibration heats up your sexual flow, and the energy of your cells allows your eggs to release. If you cannot think of a positive thought to override that emotional instability, you will become pregnant. The numbers – or codes – of the Collective Consciousness step back into your life again here in regard to how you are able to confront the issues that are presented to you. The egg swells and multiplies, depending on the consequences that you have in regard to attending to your thoughts (i.e., where you birth twins, triplets, etc.) The excuses you allowed yourself to inherit in order for you to become pregnant are what will allow the child(ren) to grow in your image. Each pregnancy is conceived in the female form, and, through the forward association and contradiction of the woman's thoughts, we predict whether that child will be male or female. Through this continuous argument that we relay back and forth between both hemispheres of our brain, we begin to understand the "Temple of the Collective Consciousness" and its responsibility as to how those thoughts construe into a fixation of a "Helical Probability" – that is, a "thought that begins to spiral through you creating your next probability". This equation conforms to a standard through a mathematical adjustment of the controlling thought. That mathematical adjustment is the end result of a woman's instability, which, in turn, promotes the gender of the child. You are not birthing yourself; you are collapsing in on yourself.

That child inherits your weaknesses and strengths, and, in a sense, this is what we call "reincarnation". The child's responsibility is to then live your weaknesses and strengths, to carry your life forward, through the best of his/her ability. When you accept this explanation, it will help you understand your children to a greater benefit. This places the onus of your responsibility back on to you, where your child must live the responsibilities that you failed to face up to within yourself at the time of gestation. I do not advise anyone not to "fall" pregnant; that is your freedom of choice. Thank you for reading these last few paragraphs; hopefully, through this information being reimbursed back to you, you can fully understand your genetic inheritance.

Now hear and understand this next announcement: A woman

with a balanced mind cannot "fall" pregnant. She would have great difficulty in trying to conceive with a balanced mind. I am not saying that it is a mistake to have children. What I am saying is that when women allow themselves to "fall" pregnant, it is through the results of their innocence collapsing in on their own understanding to themselves. They have innocently sacrificed to their relationship. Isn't this how we came into being human in the first place, realizing now that our planet is so heavily overpopulated? Many women have come to me asking why they cannot conceive; when the story is related back to them regarding their thoughts and the constituency they uphold, through rearranging their mind, the pregnancy appears.

I remember back to when I had my first two children; my first was a girl, and my second was a boy. When the family had come together one Christmas, my uncle said to me, "What a gift you have brought forth for all of us to love! You have been given your pigeon pair. Your family is now complete." The pigeon, through the Shamanistic language, is the messenger. I did not understand the message at that time, and I went on to have three more children.

Again, I refer back to Genesis 3:16, when God spoke to Eve in the Garden of Eden, "Unto the woman, he said, 'I will greatly multiply thy sorrow and thy conception; in sorrow thou shalt bring forth more children; and thy desire shall be to thy husband, and he shall rule over thee.'" Now we are beginning to understand these hidden Laws of God.

Allow me to write that passage through my own interpretation of the Metaphysical language. Unto your subconscious – or emotional mind – I will greatly multiply your grief through your innocence of understanding these thoughts; for you to come to your own decisions; and, through this grief, you shall learn to balance and eternally release your ideas; and your yearning shall give you your strength, and you shall learn to reign over yourself.

Your Notes:

CHAPTER EIGHT

To Conceive Or Not To Conceive

A woman, who is unhappy in her marriage, will usually become very disappointed when she finds that she can't conceive. The basic problem is that she is becoming dissatisfied with herself regarding her marriage; but, the reality of it is, that no children are forthcoming because of what she has attained for herself. Through her past inheritance, the genetics of the family tribe have already acquired a balanced mind.

On the other hand, if the male isn't able to father children, that means it is time for his continuation of the family line to come to the "order of his court". It is exactly the same as an animal becoming extinct; so, too, do our tribes die out. Either that man's tribe has completed its own fulfilment, or they are creating so many dilemmas through their tribal law that they are automatically cut out.

One of my patients had a very low sperm count; he was losing his positive semen through urination and leaving the dead ones behind. His wife still wanted to birth her own child, and so they kept on trying for many years. Nothing worked until I informed him that he was still living in his past, which was holding him back into his childish attitude. Through the detriment of his excuses to himself, he did not want to expand his own consequences. He was going to have to grow up and stop using the same excuses as to how he was over controlling himself.

I explained my teachings gently to both of them in order for them to be able to register what I said, and that gave them the opportunity to communicate and share with one another. The roles were reversed; they learned to understand why they had come together to form a relationship. She found that she had the power that he needed, and he found that he had the emotions she required for her pregnancy. I am happy to tell you that they have recently birthed their first child, and they are extremely happy with one another. That little boy is soon to have a baby brother, and both children will grow up in a loving household. Do you understand now why she conceived two male children?

When both partners are on the same level of their collective strength, no more children will be forthcoming. They have become justified with one another through their Divine equality. We see this way of progressive thought becoming more advanced, if we look at the current generation who are of child-bearing age.

If the man is not strong enough for the woman, it is he who promotes the pregnancy, and she then feels obligated; at that time, his power is undermined by hers. When her power is undermined by his, she creates the pregnancy herself. To put this another way, we make excuses for one another when we are inhibited through not accepting the responsibility for speaking up and declaring our truth to one another. Don't forget that our children are only on loan to us, according to - The Prophet - that amazingly precious little book by Khalil Gibran.

It is surprising how many women turn their nose up at eating meat when they first become pregnant. That is their way of apologizing to themselves for their own primordial thinking. They are tuning into the vibrations coming down through their system from the unconscious mind, in regard to the excuse they made through their intelligence endeavouring to explain to them the misconception of their thoughts.

I would like to add a brief statement here about why the late Holy Father, Pope John Paul II, had his priority right to speak his truth against abortion and the birth control pill. How can we, the human race, keep on deceiving ourselves through our innocence – or maybe it is our ignorance? How can we learn this basic rule of the Collective Consciousness – which is what we refer to as God – that, as we think, so shall we create? When are we going to stop making excuses? We invented the birth control pill nearly sixty years ago, and we still have not accepted that what we sow, so shall we reap!

Yes, the creator – or the laws of creation – has given us a hard task to deal with here, as to how each individual must be accountable to accept their right to stand to attention and be countered – that is, to accept their own truth. As we humans each evolve intellectually, we will gather into our intellectual tribe and learn to support one another through time; we shall find the courage to overcome the overpopulation in overburdened countries. If this information is brought to your attention now, the doorway can swing wide open; that doorway has an entrance of intellectual light that you can walk towards and work with for the benefit of the whole planet. It is worth thinking about.

Your Notes:

CHAPTER NINE

The Journey As A Woman

Our journey through menstruation, as a woman, is to explain to us the reasons and responsibilities regarding our role as the nurturer; it is a sacred time for the preparation of rebirthing the mind, and so we release the flow of blood. This shedding of the uterine lining equates itself mathematically through our thoughts, which have become overburdened. The heavier the period we have, the more emotionally bound up we have become. The lighter the period, is periodically created through an imbalance of hormone levels, especially estrogen, which can be rectified through medication. As our menstruation expels itself, it automatically releases the body temperature that collects through our choked-off emotions. That bleed is an automatic cleanse of every cell in the body. During this sacred time, a woman has the opportunity to refurbish her thoughts and bring her thinking back into a constituency where her personalities have the chance to realign with one another, which will support her as she moves intellectually forward.

Ovulation occurs around fourteen days after menstruation, and, if you are not thinking with a balanced mind, you have the opportunity to become pregnant at that time. That is why it is so important to release those thoughts that are no longer supporting you. The ovulation period lasts for around three days, and, once the egg is expelled, your energy closes up and brings you up into your next expedient strength, ready for the next experience to birth itself. Again, I return you back into the codes.

Many women have pain just before the time of menstruation, and so they sink deeper into their loneliness. That loneliness has been building up on their excuses over many years, and it is already creating the next month to be the same. When we do not receive the satisfaction, we are searching for, our emotions become clogged. It is an innate yearning, an innate crying, which is an inner natural manner searching for its own contentment. It is an extension as to what has been previously written, where we create our own period pain through holding onto the records of our past.

When your period is not functioning correctly, ask yourself why you need to hang on to yesterday's thinking through your lack of trust in self! Ask yourself why you need to keep up the pretence or sacrifice. Look at whether the sacrifice is for you or for your partner. If it is for your partner, stop worrying about him – come back into you and achieve your own contentment for yourself. Thousands of women have this difficulty; all of you have envisaged the same excuses. Create more time for yourself, try to let go of yesterday's thinking, and come back into accepting this God-given moment as the best moment of your life.

A few years ago, I conducted a seminar in Europe explaining the importance of menstruation; we were hoping for around fifty participants to attend. Imagine our surprise when hundreds of women turned up, where even the standing room and isles had disappeared. There were over fourteen countries present in the room. It was a long, drawn-out affair, as the languages had to be interpreted and respoken.   I was amazed at the women who just stood up voluntarily and relayed the messages into their language for those who could not understand my interpretations, and, as always, I had to remind myself of the last word that I had spoken in order to remember what sentence I was explaining to them. Most were from the medical establishments, and some had travelled from as far away as Romania, Bulgaria, Turkey, and Georgia, spending three to five days on buses, trains, and cars, even horse drawn vehicles, in order to be there.

Women are completing their menopause at a much earlier age today than in the past; this is through today's women standing more in their wealth of intelligence and using their sexual energy to create their own fulfilment.

Sixty years before the end of the second millennium, the Second World War opened a doorway for women to change, and, through their respect for others, they became more independent. Women are not sacrificing themselves now like their mothers and grandmothers did. Their breasts are getting smaller, too, and small breasts mean that those women have collected an inner strength that they use as a barrier to support themselves. Big breasts mean that those women are holding back and spending their time in service to others, where they automatically become a sacrifice to self.

In 1985, during the time I was learning tribal law with the Pitjanjatjarra tribe in Central Australia, I had a total hysterectomy that had been created through my having acute endometriosis. Endometriosis is realized through an inner crying – through lack of self-love and a lack of trust in self as a result of not being able to achieve and accomplish sexual fulfilment. In other words, that dis-ease is free to create itself within us when we are too busy bowing to our partner and not reimbursing the bow back to self. Now can you understand how the endometrial cells collect and build up when we are not reimbursing to our self?

In 1991, my old world had finished, my new world was in abeyance, and I had begun to accept my inner intellectual awakening; one morning, I awoke to find that I had haemorrhaged all over the bed sheets. I automatically checked my body, but I could find no reason for this amount of bleeding. I was totally confused, as I had thought I was living my ultimate moment.

I bled for three days, thinking that it was just something releasing itself. Then, twenty-eight days later, I started to bleed again for another three days. That bleeding has continued every twenty-eight days to this day, even though I have no womb, ovaries, or fallopian tubes. My eggs now manifest in my astral bodies, through the advancement of my spiritual education.

So where does this take humanity's earnings? What are the possibilities for the future to this never-ending story that we can create for mankind and ourselves? Think about it! Where does this redesign the future of our free will?

Your Notes:

CHAPTER TEN

Sexuality Has A Darker Side

We are all aware that sexuality also has a darker side to present to us. Have you ever realized that every woman on this planet, who has been molested or raped, has unconsciously called that rape to herself through her thinking? I know for some of you, it is quite a shock to read these words, as it was for me when I first heard of this teaching and spent many a tortuous month releasing the Collective of the codes.

You may have great difficulty in accepting and understanding that the act of rape is also a plan that God has placed throughout the mathematics for us; I ask you to please find the confidence within to look at the science of this behaviour before you read on. It was a massive learning for me to unravel the codes regarding the collection of thoughts needed to create incest. We must remember that our fear, as well as our expectations, creates our reality. I have had to listen to many hundreds of stories in order to be able to help my clients understand the hidden laws of how this act was placed before them.

Please allow me explain this theory a little further. The more your fear condenses itself over an attitude that cannot balance itself, the more forceful it becomes, and then it must release out into the consciousness. That fear is then automatically attracted to a person who is spearing himself against his own sexual inhibitions.

Man is locked in through his own molestation of self, just as woman is afraid to accept the consequences of her own actions. The more we fear the inner knowing, the more we attract the outer supremacies that must deal with the situation. The mathematics of the universal laws, returns our thinking back to us so that we can conform and learn. Please remember that many men also have difficulty in feeling through an emotional response. Why is this? It is because man has his breasts between his legs, and woman has her testicles around her neck. They both relate to the same mathematics, and they equate with one another through the same purpose. Now that sounds strange, doesn't it?

Man nourishes, and woman nurtures; both create self-satisfaction and give satisfaction to one another. When a male is not balanced in his own mind, he begins to search for his opposite, who is also not balanced in hers. There is never a mistake that is not registered with and answered by the Collective.

Here is an example of the dark side of sexuality and how the original story is handed down to the next generation. I have a dear friend who was an incest victim as a child; she had been threatened and told never to speak of it in front of the family. She has attended a few of my seminars and has now found her inner strength to make the commitment to herself; she is in the process of discovering and releasing her freedom.

She related a story to me about her previous Christmas, which she had spent with all of her family. Her cousin had come up to her and asked what she had been doing, as she looked sparkling and bright and seemed so new and different. My friend said, "I am learning to understand myself for the first time in my life, and, better yet, I am learning to release a sense of freedom that I really never knew I had regarding my own thinking. I have had it locked up for so many years, and now I am being taught how to allow it to speak its own counsel. I do not have to be quiet anymore about anything that happened to me in my past. I can face it without fear."

Her cousin was interested in the conversation, so they talked for a while, and, slowly she explained the hidden fears that had been trapped for so long – fears that were now coming to the surface. She proceeded to tell her cousin the story of her experience with childhood incest.

Her cousin began to cry, and said, "My God! I was also a victim of incest, and I was not allowed to talk about it, either!' They put their arms around each other in support, and wept.

At that moment, another cousin walked into the room and asked why they both were crying. In their newly found freedom, they shared their story with her. That cousin then said, "The same thing happened to me, but I was too scared to stand up for myself!" They learned from one another that the same member of the family had molested each one of them.

Can you imagine that man in his power? He nourished and fed himself throughout his family tribe, and was hell-bent on destroying three innocent lives. They had clung to each other subconsciously for support throughout their lives, but none of them had the courage or wisdom to stand up in order to break the old mould. Those girls had to wait until they were in their forties to know that they had all hidden these secrets from their childhood from one another, and, more importantly, from themselves; they had lived identical lives. Later on, they were shocked to learn that their daughters had also been victims of incest by that same man.

Held within that story, on an unconscious level, those women had caused that same experience to happen to their daughters. If they had found the courage to free themselves from their own bondage, the incest from their family lineage would not have been carried through to the next generation. He is now safely behind bars, and the judge, shocked by the story, was not lenient with his sentence.

Your Notes:

CHAPTER ELEVEN

Veterans Of War

One of the hardest lessons for me was listening to the "war stories" of women from many different countries where I have conducted my seminars. Here I refer to the elderly women who were alone for years waiting for their husbands to return from the Second World War, which occurred in nearly all countries. Both husband and wife had grown apart through the separation of the years away from each other, and so, upon his return, the marriage had to be consummated again.

Many women became afraid of the unnatural force that the men showered upon them; the men seemed to show so much anger through their sexual act. These women spoke of the disappointment they had felt against their femininity, which for years had been free, and they felt that they were being raped of the freedom that they had earned.

The men had come home from the war with bitter and warped emotions – and a wrenched heart that was desperately yearning for them to reclaim and try to retain their inner peace. The women watched as their men tossed and turned in their sleep, trying to return to a normal life. It did not matter which country fought which other country; I have listened, again and again, to the same story of the games we play. This story is the same told from all sides: It took both husband and wife, years to adjust and bring themselves back into the relationship that once was.

I salute those women for having the patience to understand the trauma that their men had been through. I have heard the same story from the Vietnam War veterans, and now the young ones are coming to me and explaining the same story through the wars in Afghanistan and Iraq. Is this what life on this wonderful planet is all about? Is this what we are here to acclaim? Are all these stories a precursor to represent a sense of healing for the results of war? That war is supposed to create a doorway to freedom; it is ridiculous, isn't it?

The mathematical codes to the word "WAR" is explaining to us that it is through us gaining our WISDOM that we ASCEND and RELEASE!

Your Notes:

CHAPTER TWELVE

Time For Sex

Having sex with their partner makes men feel alive; and, if they feel alive, they feel loved – and from love comes contentment. Sex is also the great manipulator; i.e., when we have an argument with our partner, the first thing we do is to stop the sex. Sometimes women feel oppressed by men, so we use our sexual power to deprive them of self-satisfaction. I had a client whose husband had run away with a sixteen-year-old girl, and our first session together went something like this:

Omni: How much time per day did you share with one another?
Client: Me? But you do not understand! My husband ran away with a sixteen-year-old girl!
Omni: Yes, I heard you tell me that, but how much time did you give of yourself to your husband each day?
Client: I did not get home from work till 10:30 p.m., and, when I did, he was in bed asleep.
Omni: How long has this work schedule been going on?
Client: For fourteen years.
Omni: When do you have time to touch, share, or enjoy each other?
Client: Sex? We do not have sex, if that is what you mean. There is never any time; I am too busy trying to earn money to keep the family afloat.
Omni: So, explain to me now, why your husband ran away with a sixteen-year-old girl? You were treating him as a child through the discourse of lecturing to reach your own satisfaction. You became the older woman, so he gladly reversed his mind and searched for a younger one.

When did that couple have time for one another? Who was carrying whom? I know that I sound very dictatorial, but so many of us get so caught up with a continuing moment through not being able to see ahead of the game. In fact, we are creating an enactment, we are not even acknowledging to ourself the game that we are participating in! We don't have an inkling that will show us what we are creating for our future learning. Both of them had created a ménage where they were focused on the one subject; there was no give and take! She was angry that she'd spent years running the household, and also having to go out at night to help supplement the wages; he was angry that she was never at home to share with him. The egos of both were in contradiction to one another, and the laws of natural attention began to work out how one could achieve top priority to rule over the other! This same story is happening every moment, in every country, right now.

Before you begin the next lesson of God Consciousness, have a glass of water and think about what you have read. The more thoughts that are spent on realizing this awakening, through understanding the mathematics of these ancient wisdoms, the less we will see this same outcome being used in the future for someone else's excuse!

Your Notes:

CHAPTER THIRTEEN

Is Your Sexuality Manipulating Your Spirituality?

Sexual satisfaction does not mean that you must have a partner; it can be just an added support to benefit you. You are quite able of achieving, all by yourself, the orgasm that will connect you to the Collective! If you have a partner, that is perfect; although, if you do not, it is still perfect! The orgasm or ejaculation that is quietly collecting throughout your body is a natural selection of endorphins that have created themselves on your behalf; they have released to remind you of the thoughts you hold under stress – that is, the thoughts that you have not allowed yourself the time to digest and release.

This equation has collected through your ego stepping on top of itself and pinning you down. In a way, it is a sense of bastardizing the emotional mind – or right brain. The difficulty is that the majority of us have been brought up to believe that the orgasm is not a healthy act. Sixty years ago, when I was a child, it was the first doorway to mental abuse, which would retard the mind as we children grew up! The subject today is no longer hidden behind closed doors, so let's bring it out into the light of the sun in order to understand and acknowledge how the situation began in the first place. It is all through your ego restraining your emotional self; it is like Father locking mother out of her own home!

An orgasm or ejaculation that you achieve by yourself is exactly the same as the one you achieve through sexual copulation with a partner. Why? Please realize, you are creating both empathies – i.e., with or without a partner – and the energy that has collected in your body is a present for you, a gift to keep you in your own presence.

The difference is that, when you are alone, the inner light that reflects back through you grows, and so it can help you come to a realization of the potentialities which you can achieve towards your next goal. When you achieve the state of orgasm, every cell in your body is walking into its own light through releasing the built - up pressure within you, so relax and make it last. As you travel in your mind with the orgasm, you can extend the feeling for hours, through continually loving yourself in that moment. While you are achieving an orgasm, allow your emotional mind to set you free.

If you feel fear about creating your own orgasm, here is an exercise that will help you begin to release the pent-up collection of endorphins which are that fear:

- Begin by thanking the sacred area of your vagina/penis.
- Close your eyes.
- Place your left hand on your vagina/penis, and your right hand on your third eye. Do this for two minutes.
- Change hands, placing your right hand on your vagina/ penis, and your left hand on your third eye. Do this for two minutes also.

Compare how you feel with the two different positions. In what part of your body do you feel the difference – the vagina/ penis, the emotional Soul energy, or the overall effect that releases in your mind? Using your right-hand shocks your ego, reminding it that another energy is present, and it is sharing the responsibility, which could become detrimental to the ego's thinking.

When you feel that one side of your body is different from the other, you are able to understand where your ego sits with your Spirituality – that is, how your ego faces up to viewing its own responsibility. If your sexuality is manipulating your Spirituality, the left side of your body is stronger, and you will find that it wants to continue to overpower your emotions. If your Spirituality is stronger than your sexuality, the language of your body automatically changes, and the right side is stronger.

By doing the exercise that I explained above, you will accept that your orgasm or ejaculation will enhance your body through rebalancing both your left and right brain. It is an ideal exercise to release the tension that collects, and it will allow the unconscious mind to step in and release those previous memories that you have had under your control. It is best to do this exercise when you go to bed at night, and you should continue with it until your vagina/penis begins to release and unfold its own control over you. Your sexuality is the doorway to your Spirituality, and each will balance and enhance the other, once we understand that the laws of our Collective Consciousness are continually spiralling energies that tune in to one another.

When next you have sex with a partner, notice where you like him/her to be in relation to your own body. Is he/she on your left or right side? Which is more comfortable for you during intercourse? Are you giving to, or receiving from, your partner?

When a woman turns to her left to face her man, she is taking the assertive roll, which means that she wants to empty her own feelings and take control of the sexual act. When she is facing him on her right side, she is lying in submission and sacrificing to him. Through a study that was conducted in the early '90s, we noticed that more women "fell" pregnant when the man was on her right than when he was on her left.

You realize now that I have given many directions in regard to the word "sex" and its involvement with your Spirituality, as the two - go hand-in-hand. Throughout all these pages, you will find quotes regarding the hidden language of your body; these quotes are there to help you recognize your deep-seated yearning to realize the magnificence that you innocently know comes through the culmination of the sexual act. It always seems to be just out of reach – or just around the corner – for some of you. Why is this so? When we try to make a success of it, the ego flusters and blunders its way through, and, in your innocence, you always feel the underlying fear that you have not fully accomplished what you are reaching up for; in other words, you are complying to act in accordance to his request. Through deciphering these hidden codes and understanding the make-up of the human mind, you can form your own opinion as to what you are searching for, and then you can release or realize the experience of the creator's gift.

When you enter into a union with another, both your and your partner's hierarchical minds consent to open your hearts to each other, and this flow of energy automatically lifts you up beyond your three-dimensional mind. Through the levitation of your mind, you are carried up into the fourth dimension, and, as you know by now, this is the entrance to the home of your unconscious mind. It is in this home that your heart and mind are in unison, which releases permanence into your enlightenment.

You now have the ability to transcend your thoughts; this wonderful word "transcend" means "to allow the ability of your mind to go beyond your own barriers and enter up into the mythical kingdom of heaven". Heaven is right here inside you, so reach for the stars that you create – these stars are created through your brain measuring your thoughts, it is an inner language that cohabitates within you and, if you are open and ready to receive, enlightenment becomes yours.

Now let us say, "thank you for the information", and move on from this subject.

Your Notes:

CHAPTER FOURTEEN

Hercules And Our Sexual Intelligence

Let's take a walk down memory lane, and I will explain a story of the past to you. I feel some of you are becoming irritated with these emotional bondages that I am releasing, so let me announce another theory of the "Big Bang" journey from female to male to you. Please remember, this book is explaining to you the Collective that is mathematically delivered to us from the unconscious mind. Up here in this Divine realm of intelligence, we cannot hide or protect one thought from another. So, let your sentences become advantageous.

The "Big Bang" creates dust and particles that magnetically attract to one another through sexual thought – all of which is what created our consciousness in the first place. Then, in order to be able to group the emotions together, we had to form a desired balance. Man and woman came onto the scene, and their unbalanced mind created the tribes.

We know that the first thought of a pregnancy is created female, and we are aware that it is the strength of the mother's overtone that determines the result of what the child must become – that is, male or female.

The vagina gathers itself into the natural orbital spin of the spiral. When it spins clockwise, the energy releases out from the spiral, and the opening of the vagina emerges. When it spins anticlockwise, the energy gathers up into the spiral, returning within the clitoris, through the vagina releasing pent-up emotions. (Remember that the clitoris, not the vagina, is comparable to the penis.) It naturally empowers itself, and the vagina reseals and closes up.

An earlier explanation of this process was created through the myth of Hercules, as most myths are in relationship to our sexual intelligence. This first "Kingdom of God" must learn to confront its own issues and face up to its own responsibilities, as this is the beginning of our transformation to reach up into our balanced mind. So, allow me explain the story of Hercules through the transformation of the Metaphysical language.

The English language has changed the name "Hercules" from its first pronunciation through the ancient manuscript of "He-rah-ark-elles". We can now begin to see the next interpretation of this story to "HE-Rah-Ark-Cells".

Let me interpret that for you: "the heavenly energy of the Rah, our inner light, is arching its way through the cells".

Whilst I was studying the ancient laws in Athens in Greece, I heard many different versions of this famous myth. Each person who told me their version of this story vowed that theirs was the "right one". The explanation of this story all depended on the intelligence of the speaker, who was interpreting his/her own intellectual mind. There are many different levels or layers, to our intellect, therefore, the level or layer, that you are releasing determines the way in which the unconscious mind reports – or reflects – back to you. As a result, each explanation was different, which allows us to see how the myths were retold through the different personalities of each refrainment. (The dictionary will insist that the word is "refrain", so I will interpret this for you.) Refrainment means "the recurring lines of a song", or "handed down through generations of humanity". (Note the Songs of Solomon in the Bible, which represent the gift we return back to our Higher Self.)

Upon my return home, I went to my computer to enter all these stories. As I typed, I noticed that I was switching from one myth/legend to another and seemingly getting nowhere. My students advised me to go onto the Internet, where I would find many different explanations, and then I could assess in my own mind which one was applicable to me. (I just love this new directional education we have available to us, which, through the computer, enables us to have the memory of the planet on a screen.) I discovered that the story of Hercules is still difficult to define, but allow me to interpret my version of this myth.

For us to emotionally relate to this story, we bring the

Metaphysics into the Latin (Hercules) from the Greek (Heracles or Herarkles). The Latin interpretation explains to us that he was supposedly the son of the God Jupiter and the mortal woman Alcmene. Remember the letters of the name: -HE is the heavenly energy at the crown of our head; -RAH'ARK is realigning our attitude, so that we may ark, ourselves up into the kingdom of God; -LES is representing the emotional minds. I will remind you that the word "ELLE" is representing both masculine and feminine energy: EL is masculine, and LE is feminine.

The difference, through the Latin explanation, is where they have added the planetary conditions, which introduces us to the story through the laws of Astrology; this inheritance was added to the original story many years ago (i.e., by the Romans). The name needs more defining to explain the difference of interpretation from the Greek to the Latin. Hercules, through the syllables of the ancient language, is pronounced "He-Rah'Ark-U-Les". So we can see that the difference between the Greek and Latin names is the letter u, which, through the codes of the Sacred Alphabet, interprets as "understanding on an inner level".

Other changes to the story occur throughout the Latin explanation: The Greek God, Zeus, becomes the Roman God, Jupiter; both were Gods of light (i.e., the sky, the lightning, and the thunderbolt), so the father of Hercules essentially remains the same in both versions. Alcmene is the mother of Hercules in both versions; translated through the codes, her name is the word "alchemy", which means the "chemistry of the brain".

I will return to the Greek version of the story. The Greeks originally took their pronunciation from Egypt, as they learned to understand the hieroglyphic explanation, and they said that Heracles was born to Zeus and Alcmene. Through the principles of Egypt, the name is the "Head of the Rah" – Heracles ("Hera-cells") – or, when we reverse it, the "cells of Hera" (the Goddess Hera is the wife of the God Zeus).

Heracles was born a twin (his brother's name was Iphicles). He grew up a rebellious child who wanted his own way. The

Goddess Hera, jealous of these twins, wanted them eradicated, as they would push her further back into iniquity, where she would lose her command over others. And so, one night after their mother had put the twins to bed, she placed two serpents in the room where the infants slept, hoping to destroy them. Let's step into the inner language of Metaphysics in order to explain that the two serpents represent the hemispheres of the brain; one serpent is the left, and the other is the right. Now we can understand that this is our lower emotional mind – that is, the one that does not wish to relinquish the power of the moment, in order to allow the next positive thought to come through.

The evolution of the Pharaoh depicts this in the hieroglyphs, where the twin serpents come out through the forehead (third eye); this coded reference explains the alignment of both brains learning to equalize with one another, which must happen before the ego can completely transform itself.

The symbolism of these two serpents enveloping the sword ("Soul's word") is known to us as the caduceus, which is now used as the symbol of the medical profession, representing the healing worlds.

Luckily for Hercules/Heracles, he was born with great strength, and so he was able to kill the serpents, strangling one in each hand. We realize that, symbolically, our hands represent the results of our actions. By the time Hercules was an adult, he had already killed a lion. In other words, his ego had been accounted for; however, this eventually diminished, and his pride became his forte.

As he grew up into manhood, his fame began to walk before him, which attracted the mind of the King of Thebes, who was named Kryon or Crion. This king offered his daughter, Megara, to Hercules to pay homage to his bravery in slaying the Nemean lion. So, through marrying Megara, Hercules became balanced again, and they brought forth three children (the mind of the next positive thought).

Meanwhile, Hera was still bent on destroying Hercules, and she sent madness to drive him insane. Through his insanity, he killed his wife and their three children. His mind had been destroyed through the taunting of his stepmother, and so, through killing his three children, he destroyed his next evolution of self. The three children represent each one of the Gods: "EL", "AN", "EA". Hercules then chose to distance himself – that is, to bring himself back into his previous normality.

As he regained his sanity, Hercules went to speak with the Delphic Oracle, who informed him that he would have to go into the service of King Eurystheus of Mycenae (in Greek, the "ae" is sometimes reversed, so this interprets as "my centre of 'EA'") for the next twelve years. This word takes on new meaning when I interpret the codes of the Sacred Alphabet. The word "Eurystheus" is decoded as "your inner God" or "your yearning for your Zeus" (i.e., light). King Eurystheus asked Hera for assistance, and she came down from her palace on Mount Olympus to deliver the twelve tasks – or labours – for Hercules to complete.

Now we are coming to realize why the Oracle asked Hercules to serve the King of Mycenae for twelve years. These twelve years, as explained through the ancient language, represent the awakening of the twelve strands of the DNA. These twelve tasks represent the opening of each strand, one at a time. (We can also refer to the twelve tribes of Israel in the Old Testament and the twelve Apostles of Jesus, when his name changed to Jesus Christ after becoming his own light, in the New Testament. Through the sacred codes, Christ interprets as "light", and light interprets as intellect.) This also represents the twelve months of each year. So we can see that every story is relating to exactly the same thing, and we remember that there is only one story.

Labour 1: His first task was to strangle the lion of Nemea (the "nemesis of 'EA'", which is the infliction of unavoidable punishment; today we refer to nemesis as the Oracle which releases the results of our actions back to us, also known as our Karma) and bring it back to Mycenae, ("my centre of 'EA'") as it was known to devour herds of animals, as well as human beings. The lion's lair was in an inaccessible cave (symbolically, the base of our skull) with two entrances. Hercules chose to wall up one of the entrances so that he could seize the lion and could kill it.

Through the intelligence of Metaphysics – or the matter of physics – the lion represents our pride, which comes to us through our ego's development not concurring with everything it is trying to release. In other words, he had to learn how to handle his pride. He took his pride and surrendered it to his father. The number one (1) represents the "I AM"; it is the introduction into discovering the self.

***

Labour 2: The Hydra of Lernaea was the second task that Hercules had to face. This multiheaded snake-like monster could destroy others with its breath, which killed anyone who came close to it. Hercules fired his burning arrows (resurrection to his mind) into the Hydra's lair to attract its attention, and then, as it came out, he chopped off all the heads, one at a time. However, the Hydra began to sprout two more heads for every one that Hercules severed. Therefore, his task seemed endless. He was attacked by a huge crab, which bit him on the leg at Hera's suggestion, and so he then had to kill the crab.

Hercules called a family member named Iolaos (another personality of Hercules), asking for assistance. Together, they cauterized the necks as the heads were severed so that the heads could not grow back again.

After cutting off the last remaining head, Hercules buried it, and it turned into a huge rock. Hercules then dipped his arrows into the toxin that was embedded in the blood of the Hydra, so that when he struck his enemies in the future, the arrows would maim them instantly.

To round it up, the Hydra (serpent) represents the past inheritance of self as it is forced to travel up into becoming the Collective Consciousness, which is where we unfold our intellectual education through releasing our inner wisdom. We are here on the earth to learn to open the seven seals that reveal our inner truth to our self. Opening these seven seals, or the seven churches of Asia, is what allows us to release up into everlasting life – or so says the Book of Revelations. And we must attain these seven seals one by one and step by step. These seven seals are in relationship to the seven vertebrae in the neck area; once opened, we have a clear pathway into the heavens.

The word "Hydra" ("Hi-Dragon") represents the ascension of the fear(s) that we have difficulty in overcoming; hence, the task given to Hercules. It had been embedded with the fear of our past generations, which resulted in the animosity towards the self! Each time Hercules chopped off a head with his sword, two heads grew in the place of the severed one. The only way he could eradicate those heads and prevent them from growing back was through fire, and he accomplished this through burning the stumps of their necks once the head was removed, which means that he had to resurrect them. They then disappeared through their own transformation into their new intellectual light.

The last head was immortal, and so Hercules buried it, and it turned into a rock (in some versions, he rolled a rock over the burial site). The rock represents the closing down of the left brain, which allows the right brain to take over the responsibility of the last head; thus, it could be transformed, given the freedom to move on without the ego interfering with the new growth. Also, the rock represents the brain in its innocence. A quick reminder for us to view is the saga in regards to the King Arthur story of removing the sword (the soul's word) from the stone, which is representing our uninitiated brain, our closed mind, before the inner journey of metaphysics began.

Let's look at the Egyptian Pharaoh again, with the double-headed snake (or twin snakes) coming through the forehead (third eye). We now understand that these two serpents must evolve up into the mind for each step of our transformation to equalize itself! The number two (2) represents the relationship that we form with our self.

***

Labour 3: The third task was for Hercules to catch the Golden

Stag, which lived in Oenoe, and bring it alive to Mycenae. The Golden Stag lived in the Arcadian mountains of Ceryneia, and these mountains were sacred to the Goddess Artemis. Hercules hunted the stag for a whole year, as it quickly outwitted every move he made. He finally managed to trap the animal and take it back alive to Mycenae.

The Golden Stag is the ultimate species in the animal kingdom; it is introducing us up into the royal behaviour of self. It represents the mind using the antlers to search the Cosmos for the truth of all things. Towards the end of my teachings in Europe, a beautiful young stag walked into my castle grounds from the nearby forest and learned to live with me. I knew then that I had completed the task that God had asked me to uphold; I was free to move on. The number three (3) represents your mind. Your mind is the evolution of your three Gods – "EL", "AN", "EA" – homing in through their transformation of self, where they must learn to become one mind.

***

Labour 4: The fourth task was to bring back the boar that lived on Mt Erymanthus, which was also in Arcadia. It was a fearsome and angry beast that devoured everything in its path. The task, as given to Hercules by Eurystheus, was to bring the boar back alive to Mycenae.

After many months of chasing the boar, Hercules ran the beast up to the snow-capped peak of Erymanthus, lassoing it and placing it on his shoulders. Carrying it back to Mycenae, Hercules delivered the boar to the king. Eurystheus was so frightened of the beast that he hid in a storage vessel reserved for olive oil.

The boar represents the feral wildness of the mind, which can only be captured through pushing it beyond the recognition of its own intelligence, as represented by the icy conditions. In other words, the mind was pushed outside its own boundaries, and so it lost control of itself. The number four (4) represents the word "temple". Your temple evolves through you equalizing your mind – that is, through acknowledging both your darkness and your light. Once we become aware of our temple, all our urges want to stay connected to this source forevermore, because we feel we have come home.

***

Labour 5: The fifth task presented to Hercules by Eurystheus was to clean out the Augean stables for the King of Elis, who housed the cattle. (Is this the precursor to Eli, who had to earn his own contentment?) These stables, through the laziness of the king, had never been cleaned. Hercules had to complete this task in one day. He dug a channel into the foundations of the stables, where he was able to change the course of two rivers, the Peneus and the Alpheus; as their flow flushed out the floors of the stables, the runoff deposited into the arid ground to fertilize the earth.

Cattle represent the word "contentment" through the laws of Shamanism. So his task was to repair his mind in a single day. Auge, in the German language means "eye"; therefore, the stables represent the all-seeing eye (third eye), which is situated in the lower centre of the forehead. The two rivers represent the flushing out and cleansing of both hemispheres of the brain – which represent the worlds of your conscious and subconscious mind – in order to receive the contentment that was due. We now begin to understand how the number five (5) represents the word "freedom".

***

Labour 6: Eurystheus next ordered Hercules to exterminate the Stymphalian birds that lived on Lake Stymphalia, also in Arcadia. These predators had wings of steel, and they destroyed everything in their path. The Goddess Athena stepped in to assist Hercules by presenting him with a set of bronze rattles for him to use to scare the birds out into the open. As they flew out, Hercules would be able to bring them down with his arrows that had been dipped in the toxin from the Hydra.

These birds represent the dark forces which like to hide under the veils of our unconscious mind. They represent our "alter ego", our "dark side" – or the Dark Lords. They do not have the strength to gain their own wisdom, and they prefer to live in their own fear. Hence, the steel-like wings which they use to permanently protect and guard themselves. Trapped in their childlike existence, they refuse to become the adult. The rattle is a toy that we give to young children to attract their attention. Athena gave Hercules two rattles, one for each hemisphere of the brain. Poison is acclaimed through our Collective Power believing in itself, wherein our Alchemy becomes stronger and stronger. The number six (6) represents how, through understanding our fears, we learn to master our self. Maybe we can see now why the world fears the number 666, as these digits represent learning and accepting the consequences as you birth into your own power to master your mind.

We also notice how Hercules had to come to the edge of the water to begin this next section of his journey. It wasn't the ocean; it was a lake, which explains to us that there was no flushing through the tides. The water was fixed, and so it could become stagnant – all of which relates to our thoughts becoming stagnant when we have nothing to look forward to. Hercules attained his first five tasks to earn his freedom from his sexual control; now his ego must accept the next form of education that had to open up within him. The ancient angelic creatures (birds) represent the evolved mathematics that the ego uses to confront others when these thoughts refuse to understand and release themselves.

***

Labour 7: The seventh task from Eurystheus was for Hercules to capture the bull of Crete and bring it back alive. This bull had emerged from the oceanic waves in response to a promise by Minos, the King of Crete, that he would sacrifice to Poseidon anything that came out of the sea. The bull was so magnificent that Minos could not give it up, and so he hid it amongst his herd, sacrificing another bull in its place. Poseidon, upon hearing of this, enacted his revenge by hexing the bull into its own madness, where it went insane. Hercules asked Minos for help to capture the bull. In doing so, Hercules would ride the bull as it swam through the waters, finally reaching Attica (the region surrounding the city of Mycenae).

Now the story begins to come together, and, as we read the seventh task, we can understand the wisdom of the myth in its fullness. The seventh task explains how Hercules collected the power of his ego and surrendered it to his higher mind. We note that the tasks are now extending him beyond his own boundaries, where he has to venture deeper into the unconscious. He had to cross the waters. The mention of Attica shows us that he had to bring the power of self up into the "attic" of his mind. Maybe now you can begin to understand the similarity in the biblical stories in the New Testament, where Jesus was placed on the cross and sacrificed his life for us. The reference in both stories is exactly the same. Remember that the first God "EL" was also once referred to as the Bull. Once we have learned to master the self, we are given the right to begin to release our education out to others. The number seven (7) represents the angelic or higher heavenly mind, where we have the right to evolve up into our unconscious thinking permanently.

***

Labour 8: Eurystheus next sent Hercules on a task to bring back the man- eating horses of Diomedes, the King of Thrace. Diomedes is similar to the ancient word "diamond", which is the light of the Collective that facets the personalities together. These horses (four mares) also devoured the flesh of passers-by. Hercules accomplished his task by capturing King Diomedes and feeding him to his own horses, which calmed down once they realized that their cruel master had been eradicated. And then they all faithfully followed Hercules to where he led them.

Through the codes, horses are interpreted as our Spiritual strength. We ride them, and they support us until we can accept our own strength. Thrace was an ancient area situated in the south-east corner of the Balkan Peninsula. In the ancient language, "TH" was pronounced as the letter t, so, initially, the word was pronounced as "Trace". The word trace means "to follow or discover; to track down and find". This word represents "past evidence", and it is also the name of the two side straps of the horse's harness. Have we used this word as it was pronounced in the first place? Those four man-eating mares represent the control that you have over your emotional inner strength.

So Hercules threw the "Master of the Mares" to the mares; and this represented the emotional mind that was now balanced through the harmony of self. The emotional inner strength then had the power to convert them back into their own temporal attitude. Remember that to master one's self is to bring all the personalities together through one's own self-acclaim. He then took them back to Mycenae – which represents the "Mother" or highest level of our emotional thought. The number eight (8) represents the harmonizing and balancing of both the left and right hemispheres of the brain. We can then move this number up to the next level, where it represents the word "infinity", which is where we become harmonized with the Soul – and this is also representing the next doorway, where we recognize the unconscious world.

***

Labour 9: One fine morning, Admete, the daughter of Eurystheus, asked her father if she could have the girdle of Hippolyta, who was the Queen of the Amazons; thus, this became the ninth task. Hercules requested a ship, and some versions of the story relate that the Argonauts sailed with him.

The Amazons were a group of warlike women, who only allowed their female children to live. As they grew into womanhood, they severed their right breast, so as not to obstruct their aim through their archery. The reasoning behind this little game meant that they could not nurture themselves – their ego was in total control; hence, the removal of the right breast. Their queen wore a belt (girdle) of gold, filled with precious stones, which was a gift from her father, the God Ares, whose domain was war.

At their first meeting, Hercules had to earn the trust of Hippolyta. Once again, Hera stepped in, disguised as an Amazon, and she provoked a furore between Hercules and the Amazons, which turned to war. Through the outcome, Hercules killed Hippolyta, thus acquiring her girdle and bringing it back to Eurystheus for his daughter.

The explanation of this strenuous task was for Hercules to overcome the emotional bondage that was keeping him from balancing his mind. Once he removed the girdle, which symbolically represented the lower crown, he was free to understand himself on an inner level, which, in turn, gave him the ability to act upon his own desires.

When Hera, through her own jealousy, tried to convince the Amazons that Hercules was trying to rob them of their own emotional hierarchy, they stood up to fight for their kingdom. So Hercules had to convince them that this was not his aim, and the only way he could convince these personalities was through encouraging them to accept the growth of their queen. The number nine (9) is the last of the single digits, and it reflects our inner knowledge to those who stand before us. The nine also represents the knowing of all, as it represents the death of our old worlds of thought. When we move up into our next level of intelligence in regard to the changes we have made in our life, we will feel comfortable in knowing that we have earned the next level of our inner wisdom.

Labour 10: The next task was to bring to Mycenae the oxen of Geryon located on the Island of Eurytheia. (Note the letter i in the word. This denotes to us that our intellect is brought forward to prepare us for the next challenge. This information is identically informing us of the change of spelling throughout the Bible. Each new letter brought into an old word is exemplifying to us the changes made intellectually through each story mentioned. Remember that these stories are informing us of the personalities every human has in regard to his/her own mind.)

The son of Chrysaor, who was named Geryon, owned vast herds guarded by the shepherd, Eurytion, and the two-headed dog, Orthros. Geryon's upper torso had an extension of three extra bodies with six arms and three heads. Now this one needs explaining. While researching the vast amounts of stories in regard to Hercules, I have never come across one that stated this being had extra legs. So we are aware that the lower half of his body was exactly the same as the one that he had been born with. Through the stories of us understanding this myth, we take note that all the Gods are still separated. The lower kingdoms have not yet been absorbed up into the educational inheritance. He is the keeper of oxen, which are animals that have been castrated. They can no longer bring forth their own excuses, so they plough through their existence in solidarity. Their totality relies on every thought they think! There is no extension to their program; hence, the three upper torsos.

By reading the books in this volume, you are learning to understand that, throughout the mythical agenda, we see the three minds, which, through the mathematical equation, must equate in balance and harmony with one another in order to evolve into the one Mind of God.

Helios, the sun God, offered Hercules his golden cup to sail the seas, and, as soon as he landed on the island, he killed Orthros with his club, and then destroyed Eurytion. Hercules captured the oxen and sailed away.

It sounds so simple, doesn't it? Let us look at a few clues of the hidden consciousness that most of us are still learning to understand. Remember that cattle represent contentment; thus, again, Hercules had to reclaim the contentment that was missing within himself! He had to release his inner contentment through chewing over all of his thoughts. The cow which has five stomachs, regurgitates its food over and over again, and, when all is balanced, it swallows. We call this "chewing the cud".

Now let us explain the monster Geryon. This name is pronounced "Chiorion", or "Chi-Orion", informing us of the energy of Orion, which, when decoded, relates to the Oracle intellectually releasing its own city of light! We have to realize the make-up of this being. We find a human with a normal body of two legs up to the thighs, at which point, the body breaks up into three different sections, where the top half is symbolically representing three different people.

Why? There is the lower mind of "EL"; the middle kingdom,

where we are educated, which, over the millennia, has been scribed as the God "AN"; right up to our heavenly home, which is "EA".

This monster still has the three Gods at war with one another. No transformation of the lower kingdoms of self evolving up into the next level of his intelligence has occurred. In other words, he has never accepted his own worth – or his own truth – and, therefore, he relies on all his kingdoms competing with one another in order to feel self-satisfaction.

Through the mythical collection of this story, we must remember that Hercules had to kill the two-headed dog Orthrus before he could get to Geryon. The two-headed dog, through the laws of Shamanism, represents the relationship as to how one earns loyalty to self. Let us just take a look at this word "Orthrus" – or "ORT of Horus", through the sacred language – o represents the Oracle, r represents Release, and t stands for Truth. If we have earned the number ten (10), through the Sacred Alphabet, we find that the mathematics have acknowledged the changes we have made in our life – that is, where we are asked to evolve up into the next level of our intelligence. Ten is confirming to you "I am my Soul." Our Higher Self is ready to guide us through the next task of our evolution; remember that the creator always has his arms wide open to support us when we fall.

***

Labour 11: His next onslaught was to procure the Golden Apples. We are finally coming to the second-to-last of these famous tasks, where we introduce you to the Golden Apples in the garden of the Hesperides, situated in the foothills of the Atlas Mountains (supposedly in Libya, according to the Greek myths). The three daughters of Atlas were forever trespassing in the garden, stealing the apples.

Again, Hera steps into the scene by placing a dragon with a hundred heads to guard the trees in the garden of the Hesperides, plus three young nymphs who assisted the dragon. Hercules walked the land, finally coming upon Atlas, whose own task was to hold up the heavens on his shoulders.

He asked Atlas to help and assist him get the apples, offering to take up Atlas's burden while he did so. Atlas was thrilled to have a respite from his burden, and gladly let Hercules take the weight off his shoulders! When Atlas returned, he passed the apples over to Hercules, only to find that he has been tricked into taking back the responsibility of supporting the heavens. Atlas, who thought he was free of the bondage he had committed himself to, found himself trapped in the same position again.

In the Italian language the word "Atlas" is pronounced as "Atlante", and, in the plural, as "Atlantes". Is this how we came to invent the word Atlantis? Do you understand why, in the mythical explanation of Atlantis, everything was perfect? Our Atlas is our brain. It is our city of light! Every thought that we think is collected in our consciousness; and so all of it is available for us to tune in to every second of our life. That explains why the atlas holds the map of the world. Now we can understand why Hercules asked Atlas to do the job for him. There is nothing that Atlas cannot do; he has the consciousness of all. You are on your way to discovering that the earth is your body, up to the beginning of your neck area, then once you have opened up the seven books that were clasped on the back of the book, which relate to the seven vertebrae of your neck, or the seven bands of peace throughout the Egyptian philosophies that have earned their own intelligence to be free, where your head is announced to you as your heavens; hence, the myth of supporting the heavens. (More on this as we move further into the rest of the books in this volume).

Take your time with the explanation of this task, as it represents the number of the balanced mind. Both brains are saying the same thing, and we have to be careful when we evolve into this form of intelligence with the self, so that we do not turn our conversation into an argument. This is similar to the latter chapters in the Book of Revelations! The word "Hesperides" sounds similar to a group of islands that we have named the "Hebrides". When we convert this word through the sacred language, it announces two words: "He-Brides". The first word, "he", represents the crown of the head, which is where the three Gods learn to become one; which is called our Heavenly Energy, which must always be balanced. Hesperides is a group of islands that converged together and became a larger consortium of energy – all expected to work together to become one! We all know that the word "brides" means "a group of women who announce their intension to join forces with the man in their life". I go further back into our evolution to remind you of the concubines in China; this was a group of femininity that cloistered around the emperor to support him.

As the power within us grows and becomes more pronounced, we need to be reminded that we must always keep a balanced mind. The same announcement is used with that group of islands; they have to form their own strength, and, usually, once this is accomplished, they stay detached and connect their mind as an assistant to the largest land surrounding them.

The Golden Apples represent the highest sweetness that grows on the land and that we can nourish ourselves with. The apple is one of the most sacred fruits in Shamanism; it is known to us as the "fruit of freedom". If we cut the apple in half, we have a map of the pentacle – or the five- pointed star – which is enlightening us into accepting that we are the four directions, plus our self! Everything is within all of us. The branches of the Tree of Life are always open and reaching up into the sky.

The number eleven (11) represents Jesus Christ. The language of eleven explains to us that famous wording, mentioned many times in the Bible: "I am as I am." I am a reflection of all that I am.

***

Labour 12: This last task was the most momentous of all, as Hercules had to face the place where the desecration of the sacred took place, which is where we have violated the laws of nature. He was sent deep into the underworld. He was initiated into the Eleusinian Mysteries, which is exactly what I am writing for you, my precious reader, to understand more appropriately who you are within and how you have the opportunity to accomplish your heart's desire. Once it comes through the heart, you know you are facing your truth. Eleusinian is also a former explanation of the word "illusion".

Through opening up his inner knowledge to understand the sacred language, Hercules could view, through his own respect, the Dark Lords of the underworld – and, also, those who are no longer here, which means that they can only support the past. This may require more explanation; as they did not accomplish to their own standard of education as to how they used humanity as their servant to benefit only themselves, they were kept locked into their past and could not move forward.

Hercules had descended into Hades, and yet he still had the support of two of the Gods, Athena and Hermes, who are representing both hemispheres of the brain. He needed all his strength now to support him, as he had to pass through the worlds of cunning thoughts to attract the three-headed dog, Cerberus, which guarded the underworld – the worlds of the bestial beasts still embedded in their own fear, where they tried to stop anyone from venturing up into their own constituency before them.

The task was for Hercules to bring back Cerberus, the guardian of the underworld (i.e., the ancient loyalty of self). His test was to tame the animal without using weapons, wearing only his breast plate and lion skin (pelt of the Nemean lion that he had slain in his first labour). These were his only two garments. Finally, he captured the beast and took it back to Mycenae. He had completed these twelve tasks, and so his life had entered into the eternalness. Hercules now could accept the seat of becoming a God on Mount Olympus.

At last, after twelve years and accomplishing the twelve tasks, Hercules was a free man. The story comes together at this point. Hercules destroyed two heads of the three-headed dog in order to reclaim his own loyalty. Remember that he could not use any weapons; he could only use the strength of his mind. Through the explanation of the Egyptian principles, the dog is represented to us as Anubis, known as the guardian to the ancient loyalties of the underworld, which we know is the home of the ego, so your insecurities find relief there. Your ego is in total control of everything you say and do, until you allow your wisdom to realign within yourself. The number twelve (12), once interpreted through the sacred law, denotes "I am my relationship". Similar stories throughout the myths all explain the hidden codes re: the "ode to see", (i.e., Homer's Odyssey, King Arthur, and many others all throughout my books). Please remember that these twelve tasks are representing the awakening and opening up of the twelve strands of your DNA.

You have been introduced to your inner rendition of the mythical agenda, through viewing how these stories have been introduced to us, just as the child who is told a nursery rhyme. So, too, is it for the adult who begins to enquire in regards to the self – that is, in respect to the Oracle and how we can answer our own questions. The first section, which I name "our innocence", is where all the Sacred Laws have created the inner sanctum for us to open up our seven seals – and that is the recorded history of you unravelling your DNA.

When we can understand the language of the myths – which are the stories that have been brought to our attention, to explain the thoughts of how each one of our personalities, earns the individual enlightenment necessary to become faceted into our inner kingdoms – we can learn to adjust our thinking in a more eloquent way. Next time you view an ancient Grecian vase, you will understand how these mythical stories relate to you. It's your choice to know who you are; no matter what religion you agree to participate with.

The stories are still the same! I can speak to you from the left hemisphere through my ego; or, I can speak to you from the right hemisphere, transforming you through my emotional language; or, I can balance both hemispheres, explaining the myth through the inner telescope, which is where you will have the opportunity to now view the inner science of you!

By now you should all understand these codes of the inner language; this has been a different explanation from just one of the myths of time. Each myth has been carried down to us, from generation to generation, in order to explain how our attitude has lessons to learn.

Now we come back to the beginning of the story to see how this journey of Hercules is supporting the clitoris on its journey to becoming the penis; this story is symbolically showing us how our strength collects through the arching of our cells. Let us remember that, when we can understand the language of the myths – which are the stories that have been brought to our attention explaining the languages, thoughts and worlds of our inner kingdoms – we can learn to add value to ourselves, by adjusting our thinking in a much more eloquent way. Thank you for taking your time to re this chapter. Don't forget to drink some water to flush the information through your system, where it will be on standby for you at any time in your future.

Your Notes:

CHAPTER FIFTEEN

Questions And Answers

Here is a series of questions and answers that I have collected from my Sexuality and Spirituality Seminars.

Question: After years of living alone, I recently went out with a younger man, and I thought that maybe he wanted to use me to brush up his ego.

Answer: You felt that he was using you, and this was an underlying disappointment to you. Why is this happening to you now? You have been given the opportunity to begin your life again, and, as you were about to do so, the younger partner naturally walked towards you. The child attracts the child. Nothing will work for you until you can first understand your own reality. Few relationships will last with this kind of thinking. Don't place the blame on the man; this is what you wanted to attract to yourself, so please look again at the circumstances that created this attraction in the first place, and allow yourself to have the unique experience that is still locked up inside you.

If you can't find your freedom in that answer, then let me tell you a story. Sex is the beginning of your evolution, believe it or not. It is the symbolic explanation of the initial books in the Old Testament. When you don't feel the need to have sex, it is through your mind feeling balanced and equalizing itself in the moment; and, while you are happy with that existence, all is well. When you start to walk backwards on yourself, your thinking begins to change in order to resurrect the circumstances that you are trying to re- create. If you are not paying attention to this, the "Old Testament" comes alive again, revisiting your intelligence and dragging you back into your own furore. When you push your partner away, through feeling that he/ she is inferior to you, in reality, you are turning away from yourself. When it comes to that primal energy searching for its satisfaction, you have to step "down' to enquire to your on thinking.

Question: I separated from my husband three years ago, as I felt he had suppressed me a great deal, and the trust had gone from our relationship; he had fallen in love with somebody else. I was too afraid to fall in love again, but now I feel the urge to mate; I am feeling very lonely inside. I would like to say, "Oh God! Please send me a gentle man, as I need to feel and receive only for the pleasure of my own satisfaction." Is that wrong?

Answer: No, it is not wrong. Why can't we all do that? You are now releasing your freedom, so allow this new you to push that sexual flush outside the door, and then let it become a blush. Your educated self is aware of your feelings, so ask the Universe to guide you. You are thinking all these wonderful thoughts, so now find the courage to put them out there. Many men are compatible to your energy, but, if you still have all your thinking locked up inside you, they will walk on by. Push your light out before you, and then see an image of yourself walking fifteen feet in front of you. It works. See it to create it!

Don't be afraid of the Goddess within you! Open your heart and let her out, as she has been closed down for a long time due to the lack of respect you received from your partner and also had for yourself. It is time to respect yourself again, and these new feelings will create emotional responses that you will be much more aware of this time.

***

Question: I come from an old country, where it is a cultural thing for a woman to give herself sexually, without feeling the man return love to her heart. How do I change these old memories to do it differently?

Answer: We have a very important gland in our body called the thymus gland, which is situated above the heart. If our heart is not opened to self, then that gland becomes blocked, and, over time it diminishes in its growth. Shamanically explained, this gland is here to remind us, "Thy must be true to thyself!" Sex is something you give to yourself in the moment; please try to understand that, through trying to please your partner and not yourself; through their innocence you are doing just what your foremothers did. They did not know any better. Has your partner tried to please you? Try to visualize and experience yourself receiving the sexual satisfaction you so dearly yearn to become aware of. There are millions of women out there with exactly the same problem. Believe me; I hear this all day long, and the same story is told in every land and language on the planet. I am now teaching in over 100 countries around this place we call home, with more than the same amount of spoken languages; as to how they explain their difficulties of learning to understand themselves on an inner emotional level.

Allow this emotional energy that opens the heart to come up, and practice the feeling of loving yourself for a little while. It will grow through its own accord by becoming a natural part of you. Your educated self is the light within you, so learn how to allow the time for you to listen to yourself. And then watch how your life changes for the better. You have many personalities of self (aspects of self), trapped inside you, as explained in the Book of Revelations in the Bible, that each person has 144,000 personalities that can be saved all through you learning to understand yourself. One third of this number is connected to your "sexual dictionary" so, release your thoughts, and then allow them to reach out into the heavens through your telepathic communication – which is through you opening up your inner thoughts, those that are being refused their own portal, and watch what you attract!

***

Question: I have been alone for two years. Recently, I had casual sex, and, as there was no emotion involved in the act, I felt very guilty. My previous relationship was terrible, especially regarding our sexual experiences, because I wanted satisfaction, and then I always felt like an animal after the act.

Answer: Why did you create such a guilty thought? What are you still hanging onto from the past? Why manifest guilt for an old excuse? Your emotions got caught up with your same old feelings that stem from your past. We have to reveal these old emotions to ourselves before we can feel ready to move on – and feel comfortable in doing so, by allowing them to be absolved by you. You have had the opportunity of spending two years alone in order to bring yourself forward from your past, and those years were not in vain. Believe in the new you!

The majority of humans want to go straight into another relationship before they fully digest the mistakes that were created in the previous one. Is the lesson learned when we do that? No, it is not! So, in order for you to learn, the Laws of the Universe step in to make sure that you repeat the same mistake again – and this will continue to happen until you have adjusted the mislaid frequencies of your mind. We must learn and earn so that the next step of our life can emerge – so that we can change for the better. We cannot keep on sitting in the same position; if we do, our life will very quickly come to a full stop.

***

Question: If a child is born with a disability, whose fault is it?

Answer: When a child is born with a disability, look at where the defect is in the child's body, and then reflect it back into yourself. By doing that, you will see where you have failed to live up to your own expectations. The more pronounced the disability that the child inherits, the longer it has taken to accrue down the line of the family DNA. The same story of your thought processes has been lived through many generations. By accepting this information, you will realize the results of your actions. The energy that is created from your positive thinking refurbishes back into the child, and this positive procedure will allow the child to free him/herself from the convivial (conniving of all) growths that have been inherited and created through his/her emotional mind.

May I reiterate by bringing in my shamanic knowledge by explaining through the mathematical laws of adjustment that cohabit intellectually with the strands of our DNA, as our thinking journeys up through the heart to our research station or brain, where every thought is measured and quantified towards you learning to unfold your inner truth. The first seven years of a baby's life from birth to seven years of age reiterate to the mothers thinking. The next seven years to fourteen years of age, the child reiterates to the fathers thinking. From fifteen years of age the child then learns to birth him/her self, through learning to become the wisdom warrior as an exemplified process of them becoming an adult at the age of twenty one.

***

Question: I know I should not worry about others, but I worry about my daughter. She is nine years old and calls for my attention all the time; she is so insecure in everything she does. For me, it is like walking on a razor's edge to stay focused and balanced, when my daughter needs so much attention from me.

Answer: Your daughter is representing the emotional responses that you have not come to terms with, regarding where you are directing yourself! The first thing to become aware of is that our children reflect back to us what is lacking in ourself at that time of interaction. She is reflecting back to you what is still trapped within you. Children also feel our repose when we are in our focused mind, and their natural urge is their fear of accepting their own responsibilities. Their thoughts run something like these: "Don't leave me now. Be there for me." "I want this and I want that." "I am only a little girl, Mummy, so your job is to look after me." In other words, your precious little girl just needs a little bit of stable nurturing and holding, which will help her to reinvest in herself. She also needs the telepathic communication that says, "I love you, and I'm watching over you."

While you focus your attention on other things, you are teaching your daughter that she has to learn to think and make decisions for herself. You are not detaching your love from her; you are detaching your emotional upheavals and insecurities, so that you may learn to trust your child to take more responsibilities regarding herself. If you think that you are doing the right thing, do not feel guilty. Our children are our mirror! It is time for you to take a good look inside yourself and realize what she is mirroring back to you.

***

Question: What is the role of the father in raising the children?

Answer: The father is the left brain, so he looks at how his son or daughter is going to represent the results of his world. The father's responsibility is to prepare the child from birth – to teach his son to create his own strength, and to show his daughter how to face up and find her own emotional strength. The father is the power of the relationship,(the nourisher) and the mother is the emotion (the nurturer).

When the baby cries, the father usually passes the child to the mother. Whilst the mother is wiping noses and changing nappies, the father begins to set up his own system, and says things like: "No, you can't do that." "Yes, you may borrow my tools, but make sure that they are put back and hung up in exactly where you found them or please put them in the right position." That is called discipline, and it teaches the child the advantages he is preparing from himself through the growth of his higher mind.

When a boy who reaches driving age says, "Dad, can I borrow the car?" The father has to judge whether or not he trusts himself enough to allow his son to have that car. He has to realize that he must encourage his son, step by step, to collect his own forthrightness. Ideally, if the father is happy that he has taught his son well, he will say, "Here are the keys, look after our car, and make sure you replace the petrol that you have been quite willing to use." The son knows that he also has the responsibility for that car, and so he accepts that he and the father are one. The father then loses power over the son, because they have become friends. He still has a life to live, and the son has to begin his own, so the father accepts his son as he is, and that gives them both their freedom. Oh, and here is one more added value that many fathers have shared with me. "I know that my family is my responsibility, and, as the years roll by, I think to myself, 'When is it going to be my turn? I seem to have spent my whole life working and supplying the demand that is presented to me.'"

Many millions of mothers have been left with most of the rearing and caring, and this has become their main responsibility in today's world, where they have had to become both mother and father. Much to my disappointment, times are drastically changing, and we seem to be losing the responsibility and the sense of family union.

***

Question: I have recently separated from my relationship, and I have an itch throughout my penis. I am so angry that I can't find my own inner strength to release that itch. Can you please explain the reason for this irritation?

Answer: You are trying to live in a section of your past that is of no longer of any consequence in this new moment, and your genetic inheritance or the laws of the universe are gently reminding you that, in this moment, you are the most important person in your life. Your ego is trying to redirect your thoughts back into the past; it does not want to face up to its own responsibility, where you are finding the courage to change your mind and move on! Again, let me refer back to the Bible, where we begin to understand the truth regarding the Ark of the Covenant. We make this covenant to our creator within. It is the Higher Self explaining our wisdom to us as to how we release and unfold ourselves in order for us, to open up our intelligence. Read the story in the First Book of Kings, chapter 8; it is a long story, but a beautiful explanation of how we are swept up into our Collective Power, from the first discovery of our sexuality to our rebirth into our Spirituality.

Stop creating excuses to smite thee! I have explained the word "smitten" previously, but I will remind you that "to be smitten" also means "to soil or stain oneself". The word "thee" is an old biblical reference, where we are communicating to our self – or speaking to our God within. Lay down your ego.

The first sexual thought begins at the back of the ears, in the mastoid area. It is in connection to the temple area, which is above and in front of the ears. The mastoid area is where the next thought is created to follow the current one. There is no emotional connection to self in the thoughts that are manifesting, so we begin through the bastardizing of our self! This is where we have total control over self, and, with this attitude autonomically releasing throughout the nervous system, we begin to stage a war within. That pins our ears back, where we refuse to hear ourselves think. We become aware of this attitude when we turn our attention outside of our own illusion and attack others. Forget the previous experience; it did not work for you. Allow yourself to be grateful to who you are and continue on through the experiences that you have gained.

***

Question: Why is the fertility of the semen deteriorating at this time?

Answer: We have become more aware that men are releasing more emotional intelligence during this stage of our evolution. Man has enjoyed bringing himself into a balance, and his male energy becomes trapped as he realizes that he does not have time to over control himself. The countdown is on for him to search for his emotional responses towards his old attitude, which will help him discover his truth. Sperm is a representation of the next thought. It is a turning point in his life where his intellect can release as an accompaniment to his new awareness of self. Marriage is becoming less important, and the old excuses are beginning to diminish. He is confronting the demands of his ego. He is not looking to create so many excuses; therefore, he does not need to produce the seeds that are there for him to achieve his own self-satisfaction. I salute their future thoughts!

***

Question: Who is responsible for my orgasm, my partner or me?

Answer: You are each responsible for the release of your own satisfaction. Try to come up into the heart area together; this allows each of you to feel for yourself first, and then release the feelings out to your partner.

***

Question: Throughout my life, I have felt that I could only be the real me if I went into a relationship with someone of the same sex, but I could never share those feelings with my parents. My mother was a hard-working woman with a job and a house and meals to maintain, also a staunch disciplinarian, and she was never available for me to share my feelings with. I had female friends at school with whom I shared my feelings. My father and brother were good companions to me, and they were always on my side when there were difficulties around the house. Sometimes I feel that they carried me through my childhood.

When I finished school I moved away, and thoughts of wanting a same-sex relationship continued, but, instead, after a six-month courtship, I married a nice man. At the time, I felt that it was "the right thing to do". We had what I would call a "feeble life", where there was no surge or pull of togetherness; we just settled in like brother and sister. In time, it seemed like all our get up and go had just got up and gone, and we grew further and further apart.

Then I began to hear about you and your teachings, so I came to listen, and I liked the way you explain things. You say that there is never a mistake in our life – there are only experiences – and you tell us how we can learn to gain our freedom through understanding why those experiences are placed before us. That wisdom has given me the confidence to move on and begin again.

After eight years of marriage, we finally divorced, and my ex-husband has now found another woman who makes him smile, and I am happy for them. After my divorce, I very quickly met a lovely woman, and we have been sharing our life together for the past few months.

Here is my question: I would like to know how homosexuality enters into our mind. Can you please explain what originally triggered those thoughts in me?

Answer: Goodness, this could take a while. I have mentioned

it previously in my book "Decoding Disease" when explaining AIDS. There is nothing new about homosexuality; it has been around for thousands of years. About every fifty years or so, it rears its head and becomes a "fashion statement", so to speak. It is a state of human acclaim when your intellect, having reached a part of its own perfection, then reaches up to search for its own compatibility. Allow me to take you both by the hand as we walk back into the ancient pathways of the Soul's yearnings. These pathways are how we began to form and create our own religious experiences, (re-ligio in Latin is explaining to us that we are linking or returning back into our inner self and learning just who we are) where these thoughts have triggered responses of adjustments in our emotional mind. It usually rears up and appears through every second generation, and it is known and shown as a valuable asset to those who are evolving mathematically in the mind. It will continue to do so until we have learned how it created itself through the Collective Consciousness.

Homosexuality did not begin in the ordinary peasant mind, as, at that time, our intelligence had not evolved into being able to understand the intellectual agreement that we walk into as we enter into the next instalment of our mathematical mind. Again, I explain that it took longer to bring time into the equation.

How did it begin to shape itself through the codes? It has been handed down mathematically through our previous generational thinking, and it is collected through a "selectual" form of control on behalf of one of the past parents. There is a part of this past parent's mind that he/she still had a difficulty in arranging and harmonizing, and this triggers a response that must be heralded and forwarded on to the next generation.

If either parent has earned their next evolution, but is being pulled back into the first-dimensional mind of the God "EL" through their own attitude dis-emboweling themselves, either one will lose sight of what is important to keep them moving steadfastly forward.

The ego then steps forward to gain control of the intellectual appreciation that this person has already achieved. That loss of direction stems from the fear inherited from the grandparents, and that fear goes way back in time, to the moment when the mathematics began to collect and add up through each generation. It becomes its own state of intelligence, through the intellectual advancement of the education into the wisdom of self.

Please take your time with this next paragraph and slowly notice how the mathematics began to collect the next phase. It has helped many a parent come to a realization of why their child stepped out of the family and stepped up into the arbitration of his/her own mind. The responsibility becomes the child's, and that child then has to mirror a reprieve for the parent's thinking. That reprieve becomes repressive in the child, and these thoughts suppress the child from finding an outlet for their attitude towards the parent. It quietly builds up throughout the child's glandular inheritance, where it becomes a supreme personality. Through the strength of that thought searching for self-satisfaction, it then becomes a priority right, which automatically attracts others who are of similar mind.

For a female to search for another female to create a relationship of self-endowment that she has accrued, she emotionally hides behind her father figure. Through her objection to the symbiotic suggestions of her mother's control, and also to receive the support that she is searching for, she passes on her alternated strength to her father.

For a male of the species who is looking for a homosexual relationship, it is the opposite. He protects himself by disguising himself through his mother's garments, and he looks for support from the emotional mind of his mother, through his objection to the attitude of his father. Remember that we are talking about our thoughts, which are quietly accomplishing their own desire to attain and reach a sense of freedom. In most cases, the grandmother of their family understands exactly why the offspring has chosen this style of life. Why? She has reached the peak of her own understanding through the years of her own marriage, and so she can realize through her own children's accomplishments what the grandchild has inherited.

So, to bring your question back into an alignment, we begin to see that the discourse amongst the family tribe, is the reason why people have been programmed through their generational inheritance to live out the alignment of becoming homosexual. Please remember that the Soul is neither male nor female. It is the combined energy of both brains. Once the mind has equated itself, the ego transfers its ideas and builds up a personality which becomes imperious to search for a compatibility of the same mind of self. So, the desire of the male is intellectually looking for the phi-male (female), which is the mathematical balance of himself, to create a partnership. We must also equate the balance of the subconscious energy and watch how it urges this personality up much higher into the unconscious layers of the mind and into the musical area of the Soul; this area desires a mirror image, and it attracts a loving relationship with another Soul.

Now, when it comes to the woman, we see a reversal of energy. We see how the woman is searching for the woman she has overstepped within herself, through shielding herself behind her father figure. This is where we bring the word "feminine" into the language. Let us look at the word "fem-in-in-ity". Again, it is a relationship of an intellectual arrangement that collects and nurtures itself through her intellectual balance, and on behalf of herself. Again, the subconscious mind urges the personality up into the ethereal layers of compatibility.

You would have to take the journey back through your own family's leniency towards themselves in order to see how the outcome presented itself to you. Take your time, it's on your side, I wish you well.

***

We have come to the end of this explanation of your sexual behaviour, and I would like to remind you that your sexuality is the doorway to your Spirituality. It is your lessons in understanding the truth of your inner self. This energy transfers itself up through the whole body as our intelligence awakens. The sexual act, through its desire for its own completion, is the search for the satisfaction of our Divine completeness; and so, it pleases our understanding of self-worthiness and relaxes the moment. Our primal urges have been replaced, and we feel fulfilled. The left brain has enlightened its moment, and the right brain rebalances and feels harmonized.

Sex clears and rejuvenates the seven seals, which is the doorway to us walking our own pathway into our self-discovery; through giving them the blessing they have earned through rejuvenating themselves. It is a walk, step by step, towards the opening of your Book of Revelations, which when read is so similar to the journey explained throughout the land of Egypt, also China, which is explaining to us the journey of you discovering yourself. Sex harmonizes the intellectual light in our cells, creating a brief moment of enlightenment. It makes you feel good! It allows you and your God within to become as one.

May you all inherit the wind, which we know is the breath of God, through the **Greatness** of the **Oracle** of the **Divine**.

Thank you for reading my story.

APPENDIX A
Review Of Our Individual Universal Law And The Laws Of The Universe

Introducing our Individual Universal Law and the Laws of the Universe, excerpt from my book "Decoding the Laws of the Universe".

It is our own Individual Universal Law creating the Laws of the Universe! It is where we all become involved, and, through time and cause and effect, we have created and advanced our evolution for all humanity to inherit. The Laws of the Universe, (also known as the Universal Law, the God essence and many other terminology), is the Soul Energy of the Collective Consciousness; it is a mathematical program of all that is.

It is the Soul's purpose (each person) to be here on the planet, and each Soul must release and improve the energy that has collected from the past. We are asked to live and discover this inner truth that is embedded in the depths of the Laws of the Universe, which are embedded in each one of your cells. Our journey is to repair the thoughts of our previous generations as we journey forward which expedites their layers of confinement. Please remember, we have evolved for a very special reason.

Our own Individual Universal Law refers to the metaphysical philosophy that each individual is responsible for creating their own reality through their thoughts and emotional intelligence. The nature of each person's thinking, unique perspective and energy contributes to the overall consciousness of the universe. This knowledge is transformative on a personal level; once we understand, we can make great waves for all of humanity to inherit.

OVERVIEW:

Our Individual Universal Law

We are each our own Universe with our own Individual

Universal Law, and we exist within a greater Universe that has its own proprietary law as well.

You are your own Universal Law; and, as you think, so, too, you create. You are given this gift to be in charge of how your thoughts create your world. As you allow one thought to finish itself, the next one is waiting to release itself to you. Your next thought will wait patiently until you are silent enough to allow it to come through.

Your Individual Universal Law is not created by what you do, but, rather, by your silent thoughts, regressions (thinking in the past), joys, frustrations, and peace. It is the energy and evolution of your emotional intelligence and how you connect to you.

Once you understand what your Individual Universal Law is, keep yourself focused, and you will be able to fulfil all your desires. Life will bring you up, through the temperance of your Soul, and, when you can define this inner education, you will become and join forces with the Divine.

The Laws of the Universe

It is our Individual Universal Law creating the Laws of the Universe! It is where we all become involved, and, through time and cause and effect, we have created and advanced our evolution for all humanity to inherit. These Laws of the Universe are also known as the following: Collective Consciousness, Universal Law, the God essence, Collective Library of the Consciousness, World Consciousness, Collective Inheritance, Collective Memory, Collective Mind, Collective Soul of the God Force, Akashic Hall of Records, Hall of Recognition, Soul Energy of Collective Consciousness, and my favourite, the Eternal Matrix.

The Laws of the Universe (Collective Consciousness) registers all our conscious thinking, which must return to the conscious mind in order for our energy to continue to grow through the human evolution. The past from day one, is still alive in the Collective Consciousness; that Collective Inheritance is all of our thinking and evolution. We cannot forget yesterday, but we can absorb it; we can soak it up into our own consciousness and use it in the moment.

The Laws of the Universe answers to our thinking in a balanced way, although, it is not always in the way that we expect it to be! Another name for it is Karma, or the "Kha-Rha-Mha", if we explain it correctly, for this goes back to the early language of the Armenians and the hieroglyphs of Egypt. If we pronounce it in its correctness, it is the cause and effect, or the accidental and occidental; it is the occidental that is the key to your wisdom. The occidental is the final outcome of the length of your stay on this planet. The occidental is the light that keeps this planet alive.

So, your knowledge of these secrets can carry you to the place where you have the opportunity to dance along with these Laws of the Universe.

As you begin to believe in yourself, your Soul gives you never-ending gifts of knowledge. To believe in yourself takes a tremendous amount of courage for you to release, and that courage will lead you into other parallel worlds of existence. Those worlds align within and open you up to your inner worlds, where you have earned the freedom to use them to promote your tomorrows.

EXPLAINED FURTHER—DELVING DEEPER:

Our Individual Universal Law

Let us explore further, our own Individual Universal Law. As stated previously your Individual Universal Law is not created by what you do, but, rather, by your silent thoughts, regressions (thinking in the past), joys, frustrations, and peace. It is the energy and evolution of your emotional intelligence and how you connect to you.

Understanding and connecting with our emotional intelligence is key to tapping into our Individual Universal Law. This involves becoming aware of our thoughts, of our emotions, learning to identify and process them, and understanding the ways in which they influence our actions, and outcomes we experience in life. By paying attention to the patterns and themes that emerge in our lives, we can begin to identify the underlying beliefs and values that shape our perceptions of reality.

Our emotional intelligence is instrumental to the evolution of our Individual Universal Law. Our emotions are energy in motion, and they have a vibrational frequency that attracts experiences and circumstances of a similar frequency. When we are in a positive emotional state, we are vibrating at a higher frequency, and we tend to attract positive experiences and people into our lives. Conversely, when we are in a negative emotional state, we are vibrating at a lower frequency, and we tend to attract negative experiences and people into our lives.

Therefore, to evolve our Individual Universal Law and attract more positive experiences into our lives, it is crucial to work on our emotional intelligence and maintain a positive emotional state as much as possible. This means being aware of our emotions, expressing them in healthy ways, and choosing to focus on positive emotions such as love, gratitude, joy, and a feeling of peace with oneself. We can use mindfulness, staying in the moment and have an awareness of the chatter of the mind.

You can also examine your "relationship of self". Your relationship of self is the way you relate to you. It is created by the thoughts you have about yourself, belief in self, the emotions you feel about yourself, your judgements about yourself, your perception your self-worthiness and how you honour yourself—your internal dialogue to self. When your belief in self builds upon its own strength and creates your next positive thought, your life becomes so much easier for you to manage.

How can we improve our relationship with ourselves, and what steps can we take to cultivate a more positive internal dialogue that supports our self-belief and self-worth? How can we break free from negative thought patterns and judgments about ourselves, and build a stronger foundation of self-love and self-acceptance and discipline, that empowers us to create a more fulfilling life? How can we identify and change limiting beliefs that may be holding us back, and replace them with more empowering beliefs that support our growth and development? The answer is by cultivating a positive internal dialogue. Improving our relationship with ourselves involves several steps. Firstly, we need to become aware of our current internal dialogue and how we communicate to ourselves. We can start by observing our thoughts and emotions, and noticing any patterns of negativity or self-judgment. Once we have identified these patterns, we can work on changing them by replacing negative self-talk with positive self-talk and affirmations of "I believe in myself". To cultivate a more positive internal dialogue, we can furthermore practice self-compassion and self-forgiveness. To break free from limiting beliefs and judgments about ourselves, we can challenge these beliefs and reframe them in a more positive and empowering light. This can involve seeking out new perspectives and information, and exploring new ways of thinking and being. When your belief in self builds upon its own strength and creates your next positive thought, watch how the miracles manifest in your life where you will find you are continuously working as one with the universe.

This journey is yours and cannot be given to anyone else; the responsibility is yours alone. The hierarchical mind/ unconscious mind/higher mind, also known as the Higher Self, will always be there to step in front of you, protecting and holding you firmly when you cannot believe or when you have lost your trust in you. Our Higher Self is a deeper and evolved aspect of our being and has access to higher levels of wisdom, intuition, and guidance. Our Higher Self, presents experiences for us. It gives us the opportunity for our thoughts to repeat throughout our life until we can find the strength to overcome them. This suggests that our Higher Self may be trying to teach us something or help us grow by presenting recurring negative thoughts, experiences, or fears.

Our thinking can create our fear in the moment by the way we perceive and interpret our experiences, this leads on to attracting Depression! Our thoughts and beliefs regarding a current situation can trigger a fear response in our body, even if there is no actual physical threat. Our thoughts can also create a negative feedback loop, where the fear response reinforces the negative thinking, leading to more fear and anxiety. By changing our thinking and challenging our beliefs, we can break this cycle and reduce our fear and anxiety in the moment.

If you find yourself repeatedly experiencing negative thoughts, fears, or experiences, it is important to stop them before they become greater. Remember the traffic lessons you learned in school: stop, look, and listen. Take a moment to search beyond the present moment and see how this energy or thought is recreating itself. To search beyond the present moment, is to take a step back and analyse the situation objectively.

One way to do this is to observe the thoughts and feelings that arise when the negative thought, experience or fear resurfaces. Ask yourself questions such as: What triggered this thought or feeling? What emotions am I experiencing? Is there a pattern to these thoughts and feelings? Reflect on how this thought or fear has impacted your life and try to gain insight into why it keeps coming back. This process of self-reflection can help you identify the underlying causes of the negative thought or fear and find ways to overcome it. This is not a learning experience, but an earning experience.

The difference between the two is that learning means "looking at" something, while earning means "looking through" it. Your Higher Self, presents these experiences to you as an opportunity to overcome them. One thing in life is certain: You cannot run away from yourself. There is nowhere to hide! You create your fear in the moment through your thinking. Write this down: "My fear is created by me, as I am refusing to live and accept this Divine moment in my life." By acknowledging your power over your thoughts, you can take the first step towards personal transformation.

If I can help you to understand and accept, where you can act out your thoughts through self-confidence and assurance; then we are both winners. Hopefully you will have the opportunity to rake away your fears, as this is the sole— and Soul—reason for you to be here, and it is what this life's quest is all about. We rake up all the leaves after the autumn season has ended, and we prepare the garden for winter. Winter is the time for hibernation, and it is through our own hibernation that we are given the time to dichotomize, which means to sort out right from wrong and refrain from making the same mistakes. When we look out our window again, our garden looks tidy and free; the raking has allowed it to regain its own silence and to breathe new life as it prepares to birth itself for the next season.

For years in the journey to discover this metaphysical knowledge (that is, before I became an Adept in the Secrets of the Universal Laws), I went into the "Worlds of Invisible Kingdoms" (explored other dimensions) and was asked by my teachers to read the Bible in the reverse from Revelations back to Genesis, instead of the other way around. It is not necessary for you to do this. My teachers informed me that, by doing this, I could bring through a resonance of intelligence that all of humanity could view from within themselves—where they could understand the capabilities of how their intelligence unfolds itself, and then that knowledge would be available for them to add to what they had already achieved. "Why?" I asked my teachers. "Your program fits the bill" they told me. "What program?" I persisted. "The thoughts of your previous generations have been indelibly imprinted in you, and you have made yourself available; you asked, so now you have the opportunity to receive!" That's what they told me!

To further explain, a "life program". Your life program was created through your parents' DNA, which provided the basic principles for you to become you. Your task is to unfold yourself through the disadvantages of your parents' judgment and through their innocence in (mis)understanding themselves! You have chosen to live what your parents were too afraid to face through their acceptance of self as they understood it, and, more importantly, you have also chosen to live their gains.

Your life program keeps on creating itself through each of your thoughts building upon the other, and the transformation continues until you have taken your last breath. That energy force field grows in strength and opens you up into your Higher—or heavenly—Self. That Higher Self follows you through every thought you think, always encouraging you to create and expand your thinking.

To carry your DNA inheritance into your next step of humanity's earnings is how and why you have evolved to be here, through balancing and clearing your past generations' thinking and programming the basics of the mind of your future generations. Once we have accepted this program, it is no longer a detriment to your consciousness; the freedom you create in your mind will allow your intelligence to have the ability to evolve even further. Once we have recognized and solved the tasks that have been given to us by our genetic inheritance, we are free to collect more information to add to the benefits available to us beyond this program.

During those years of my internal searching, my intelligence grew into the "Wisdom of the Sages", where I could see through the layers of restriction that I had hidden behind for my own protection. I also began to study the science behind humanity's thinking, and, as this information grew, understanding it fully became my ultimate goal; as a result, over the years, all knowledge consumed me. I found I could unite the plumber with the librarian, the lawyer with the builder, the electrician with the social worker, and then unite them all into a whole! It is the relationship of self that connects us to the energy of our total evolution. This knowledge has grown stronger and stronger over the last thirty years of my life. Subsequently, I brought all this information into a format that is ongoing in every moment of my life. I learned how to transfer this knowledge into the human body by beginning with just one cell.

Once you understand what your Individual Universal Law is, keep yourself focused, and you will be able to fulfil all your desires. To keep ourselves focused and fulfil our desires according to our Individual Universal Law, we need to maintain a clear and positive mindset. This means consistently monitoring our thoughts and redirecting any negative or limiting beliefs towards positive and empowering ones. We can do this by practicing mindfulness and being present in the moment, observing our thoughts and choosing to let go of any that do not serve us. Visualization and affirmations can also be powerful tools to help us stay focused and aligned with our desired outcomes. By visualizing ourselves already having achieved our goals and repeating positive affirmations that affirm our abilities and worthiness to receive what we desire, we can tap into the power of our Higher Self and attract more of what we want into our lives. Life will bring you up, through the temperance of your Soul, and, when you can define this inner education, you will become the Laws of the Divine.

<u>The Laws of the Universe</u>

Let us explore further The Laws of the Universe. As stated, it is our Individual Universal Law creating the Laws of the Universe! It is where we all become involved, and, through time and cause and effect, we have created and advanced our evolution for all humanity to inherit. The Laws of the Universe (Collective Consciousness) registers all our conscious thinking, which must return to the conscious mind in order for our energy to continue to grow through the human evolution. The past is still alive in the Collective Consciousness; that Collective Inheritance is all of our thinking and evolution. We cannot forget yesterday, but we can absorb it; we can soak it up into our own consciousness and use it in the moment.

The Collective Consciousness registers all our conscious thinking by storing and recording every thought, emotion, and experience in a universal database or energy field. It is the energy of the thought, emotion, and experience that registers with the Collective Consciousness on a quantum level. Basically, explained on a quantum level, our thought energy interacts with the universe through the observer effect. This effect describes how the act of observation can change the behaviour of particles and systems in the universe. When we focus our thoughts on something, we are essentially observing it with our consciousness, and this observation can affect the behaviour of particles and systems related to that thing. According to quantum physics, all particles and systems in the universe are interconnected and entangled. This means that our thoughts and intentions can have an impact on the behaviour of these interconnected particles and systems. Our thoughts and emotions emit energy waves that can influence the energy of the Laws of the Universe, the Collective Consciousness. (The physical particle-like structure of matter existing in time-space, in which it exists non-locally "encoded" as a wave frequency in the past, present and future of the Collective Consciousness—the holographic universe).

This collective inheritance of knowledge and wisdom is available to us all and can be tapped into for personal growth and evolution. (Time-space reality is the frequency domain of the Higher Mind as well as the Collective Consciousness). As individuals contribute their thoughts and experiences to the collective, the database expands and evolves, contributing to the evolution of humanity as a whole.

The Laws of the Universe answers to our thinking in a balanced way, although, it is not always in the way that we expect it to be! Another name for it is Karma, or the "Kha-Rha-Mha", if we explain it correctly, for this goes back to the early language of the Armenians and the hieroglyphs of Egypt. If we pronounce it in its correctness, it is the cause and effect, or the accidental and occidental; it is the occidental that is the key to your wisdom. The occidental is the final outcome of the length of your stay on this planet. The occidental is the light that keeps this planet alive. That gift from the All That Is, is our attainment, and it is also how we have produced our next moment. Weather patterns, dis-eases, viruses, and wars are all creations of the atmospheric conditions of the Collective Consciousness; they are the results of the thinking of this planet. Our accidents are what we have produced for ourselves through our thinking. The occidental is the explanation, as to how we have gathered and achieved the accident in the first place. It is not only what you have done to you; it is how the Laws of the Universe answer back to what you are doing to you. I like to refer to the occidental as the "messenger" represented as the Pigeon throughout the Laws of Shamanism. With its sonic sound, it homes in on a catastrophic conclusion of thought, and then it delivers the message to our heavenly home, which is our brain.

APPENDIX B
Brief Metaphysical Overview Of The Brain/ Mind/Levels of Consciousness

We have many different levels of consciousness that are available to us as we grow into our new relationship of self. As our intelligence releases itself from our bone matter, we are able to access these layers of new found "grace", which empowers our inner self, where it evolves throughout our language to reform into the word "beauty". Throughout the Laws of Shamanism, we are gifted with the species of the swan in the creation of the human brain, as this species represents the waters, (the Collective Consciousness), known to us in the beginning as the emotion, grace, where we are able to sense and feel how to slide or glide our way through the endowment of self-acclaim. We are also gifted with each species of animal, vegetable, mineral, earth, the waters or the sky (all endowed with an emotion of energy in both negative and positive form), which is created throughout the evolution of the human brain during the first three months of human gestation. We class this as the ninety-day sentience, as our brain is superseded with every species that has earned its own vocabulary to live in our domain.

Our brain has two hemispheres—two parts. The left-brain is our logic (conscious mind). The left-brain is our masculine side; our ego, our primal fear, and as stated our logic. It portrays how we are representing ourselves to others through releasing from our next thought, as it can only register thirteen words per minute. It is also known as the child within. It still has to grow and mature into the adult phase. This hemisphere only looks at! It has difficulties to look through where it can view the whole picture as in its natural form it does not have the endowed intellect to understand as it is still too afraid to take the journey into the unknown.

The right brain is our emotions (subconscious mind). The right brain is our feminine side, our inner creative language. We give out to others with the right side, where our energy in motion—or emotion—creates itself from how we are giving and receiving to and from the self. The right brain represents what we are doing to ourselves within, and what we are capable of receiving through ourselves.

The people who live in their logical ego sense are perfect, and so, too, are the people who live in their creative emotional sense. In understanding the logical sense, we understand through our primal inheritance, where it begins to fit with common sense. The mind of logic is the echo from whatever is created, and it is also, what we attract in our outer worlds; the emotional mind sits within and takes care of our sense of responsibility.

We cannot survive on this planet without both ego and emotions. Our journey is to learn how to balance both brains so that we may advance our awareness of the supportiveness of our unconscious mind or Higher Self, (also known as the supra-consciousness, higher mind, ultra consciousness etc.). The unconscious/higher mind is the freedom with which we can tune into ourselves, but only when the other two parts of our brain have balanced through our attitude to our self. The unconscious/higher mind is the highest realm of our intellect, which mathematically measures, every thought that we think (mathematically measuring the inner balance of the mind, to build-up the energy of thought. Mathematics is the equation of cause and effect).

It has taken us a few years to come to terms with the intelligence of the unconscious mind. We have always been aware of it, but we do not quite understand it. We are becoming more aware of its intellect as we open up our own intelligence with each positive inner step we take. The unconscious mind is communicating through us, twenty-four hours a day, and, slowly, we are becoming aware of the advanced language of how it communicates back to us.

If we like to take this further, our left-brain, our conscious self, is firstly recognised as the child within, it is responsible for the first and second-dimensional mind. Our right brain, our subconscious self; is responsible for the third dimension and the relationship to the introduction into the fourth dimension, which relates to time. The balance of both brains through looking into one another, is when we enter into the doorway which delivers us up into our unconscious mind, which allows it to be responsible for the "temple of self" where we have earned the responsibility to live up to its expectations. Temple of self means we are training our self, moment by moment, to have control over our thinking. Our unconscious/higher mind is the make-up of our Divine Inheritance—or the Language of our Soul—it is when we have earned our spiritual life force. The unconscious/higher mind is the world of telepathic communication.

Books By O.M. Kelly (Omni)

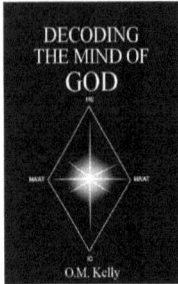

Decoding The Mind Of God

Author O.M. Kelly's seminal work, "Decoding the Mind of God", is a compilation of nine volumes of metaphysical information based on the research into the coded information of the Laws of the Universe, also known as the Collective Consciousness, and represents a groundbreaking contribution to our understanding of the metaphysical universe. Now, all nine volumes are being released as separate, revised books, each offering a unique perspective on the universe's workings. Omni's work has been widely acclaimed for its depth of insight, and her contributions to the field of metaphysics have been groundbreaking.

The nine separate volumes encompassing:

The Laws of the Universe
Thought
Dis-Ease
Death
Sexuality and Spirituality
The Dolphin's Breath
Sacred Alphabet and Numerology
Sacred Fung Shwa
Extra-Terrestrial Intelligence.
Updated version of each book now being released separately.

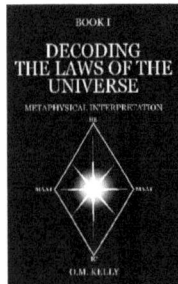

Book I. Decoding The Laws Of The Universe

If you're looking to unlock the hidden potential within you and transform your life, "Decoding the Laws of the Universe" is the book for you. This powerful and insightful book is designed to help you understand the deeper, metaphysical aspects of life and tap into the transformative power of the universe utilising the secrets of our Individual Universal Law.

This book serves to introduce you into the secrets of our Individual Universal Law. This amazing knowledge and wisdom, is transformative on a personal level and creates the opportunity for you to interrelate with the Laws of the Universe. Throughout this book, you will dive deep into the inner workings of your mind and discover the hidden laws that govern your life. You will learn about the alchemy of the mind and how to harness its power to create positive change in your life and the world around you. Through the lens of Metaphysical philosophy, you will gain a new perspective on the world and your place in it. You will learn how the universe communicates with you through coded intelligence and how to unlock the hidden messages that are all around you.

This book is a journey for personal transformation and spiritual growth. Take a voyage of exploration of the expansive vistas of information discovering the codes of Metaphysics and the Quest of Life. You will learn the Metaphysical coded wisdom of the ancients for the necessary mind elements to transit into a higher mindset. Explore the secret relationship between the Earth and human beings, the higher mind, the Metaphysical journey, the importance of self, belief in self, the codes of mythology, a higher level of attainment, releasing the past, fears and evolving one's light on a Metaphysical level, what causes stress, work place promotion and why it does not happen, and many other topics. Included is a short overview of the conventional Twelve Laws of the Universe.

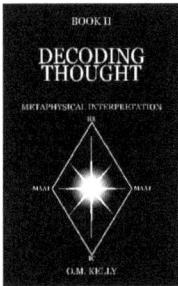

Book II. Decoding Thought
Welcome to a journey of self-discovery and exploration of the mysteries of the universe. "Decoding Thought" is a ground-breaking book that explores the power of the mind and the principles of metaphysical thought. Through a deep exploration of the mind and body connection, the author provides readers with insights to unlock the full potential of their thoughts. This book provides a guide to harnessing the power of the mind to create the life you desire. With explanations of metaphysical principles, the book makes these often complex concepts accessible to readers. "Decoding Thought" takes you on a journey through the vast landscape of the human mind. Explore the mysteries of thought power, and how it can shape our reality and transform our lives. The power of thought is not just a theoretical concept. It is a tangible force that can be harnessed to bring about significant changes in our lives.

This book can expand your consciousness and open your mind to new possibilities. By exploring the metaphysical principles that underlie our existence, you can gain a new perspective on life and the world around you. This book provides through a metaphysical interpretation explanations into the various aspects of thought power, including how it is linked to our DNA, and the roles played by the pituitary and pineal glands in our thought processes. O.M. Kelly also explains the metaphysical language in reference to the codes of the Egyptian Philosophies, the Bible, myths, cultures, and how they connect to the power of thought. The journey continues with a deep dive into the inner Secret School of Metaphysics, where we discover the Alchemy of the Brain and the pathway to our truth. Discover the unconscious/higher mind, and our Life Quest, which opens the doors to the Psychometric Consciousness. Through the lens of metaphysical interpretation, you will gain a new perspective on the impact of thought on our mental and emotional states that includes a look at Depression, Coping with Change and how to retrain our brain patterns to be positive and moving forward for our Financial Abundance and manifesting prosperity. The book ends with a brief overview of the brain/mind, and a short Q&A on thought power. This metaphysical book on the power of thought is a guide to discovering your true potential and creating the life you desire.

"Decoding Thought" is a must-read for anyone seeking to unlock the full potential of their mind and harness the power of the universe to create a life of fulfilment and this book serves as an invaluable resource.

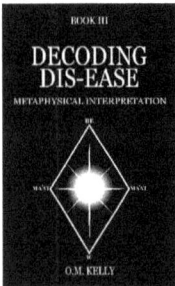

Book III. Decoding Dis-Ease

Introducing "Decoding Dis-Ease" a Metaphysical Interpretation into understanding the intricate web of factors that contribute to our health and well-being. From the author of several groundbreaking works on the interaction of the mind and body, this book delves into a wide range of topics related to dis-ease. It is a fascinating and insightful book that offers a fresh perspective on health and healing. It is a must-read for anyone interested in the mind-body connection.

Readers will be inspired to embark on a quest of discovering the codes within themselves, recognizing that every cell in our body is pure Cosmic Consciousness. They will also gain a deeper understanding of specific health topics such as the thyroid, the kidneys, men's problems, and many other topics from a Metaphysical perspective. The book also examines how a dis-ease is given to us in group energy and the complex interplay between our bodies and minds, and how every human has the consequences of all that we do and experience.

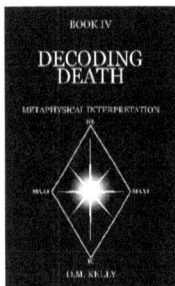

Book IV. Decoding Death

Looking for a thought-provoking exploration of death and the afterlife? Look no further than O.M. Kelly's book, "Decoding Death".

"Decoding Death takes us on a transformative Metaphysical journey through the mysteries of the Universe. O.M. Kelly—known as Omni—provides an expanded horizon of possibilities, awareness, and a transformative perspective. In this book, Omni delves into a wide range of topics related to dying and death, from the loss of a loved one to a viewing of the afterlife. Omni has a unique ability to view the Laws of the Universe using her extraordinary state of heightened awareness and multi-dimensional perception and through the lens of metaphysics offers a unique perspective on the nature of death and what it means for the human experience.

Omni shares personal experiences and stories, including the passing of her late husband, brother, and parents, and offers a metaphysical insight for those dealing with loss and grief. She explores the transformational process of death and the potential for spiritual growth and enlightenment. The book explains that the human experience of death is part of a larger Universal process that is ultimately guided by a higher intelligence referred to as God (Laws of the Universe/Collective Consciousness) or whatever name you prefer. Omni's exploration of death is both metaphysically comprehensive and thought-provoking, offering readers a deep and nuanced understanding of one of life's greatest mysteries. With chapters on the Three Doorways—Three Stages of Death, The Quantum Hologram—Why a partner dies for the other partner to progress in the "Journey of Life", The Passing to the Afterlife, and many other enlightening chapters, "Decoding Death" offers a unique viewpoint. By drawing on a range of religious, philosophical, and metaphysical perspectives, Omni offers a compelling vision of the human experience of death and its role in the larger Universal Law.

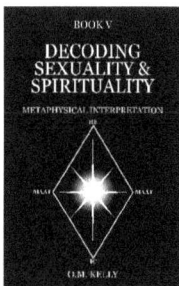

Book V. Decoding Sexuality And Spirituality

Welcome to "Decoding Sexuality and Spirituality" by O.M. Kelly. In this book, explore the fascinating relationship between our sexuality and spirituality, and how these two aspects of ourselves are intimately intertwined. Delve into the concept that sexuality is the doorway to our spirituality, and examine the powerful and transformative energy that is generated when we fully embrace our sexual selves. The book also explores the notion of the metaphysical orgasmic cloud, and how it can be used to deepen our connection to our spiritual selves. We will also examine the role of marriage in our sexual and spiritual lives.

For women, the book offers a unique perspective on the journey of embracing sexuality and spirituality, as well as insights into the different stages of life and how they impact our sexual and spiritual selves. Drawing on both ancient wisdom traditions and metaphysical mythology, the book examines the myth of Hercules and how it relates to our sexual intelligence. By decoding the symbolism of this myth, we can gain a deeper understanding of the ways in which our sexuality and spirituality intersect and influence each other. So if you are ready to embark on a journey of self-discovery and unlock the true potential of your sexual and spiritual selves, then "Decoding Sexuality and Spirituality" is the book for you.

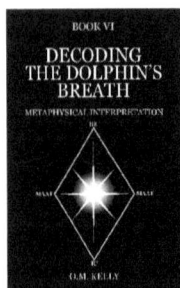

VI. Decoding The Dolphin's Breath

"Decoding The Dolphin's Breath" by O.M. Kelly (Omni) is a captivating exploration of the relationship between humans and dolphins. The book begins with a poignant account of a real-life encounter between the author and a group of wild dolphins, setting the stage for a deep dive into the spiritual and metaphysical significance of dolphins. This captivating book takes readers on a journey into the heart of the dolphin-human relationship, exploring the ways in which these majestic creatures can help us attune to the power of free will, and telepathic communication.

Throughout the Laws of Shamanism the wonderful Dolphin in consciousness, represents the attainment we can reach through ourselves earning our freedom of will. This book explains the benefits of the dolphins breath—the why and how we use the breath that influences our divine mentality. Further, it's a story which reveals how the dolphins have taught us the process to be free of fear, and to tap into the Language of Babylon—to understand the language of Earth. One of the key themes of the book is the idea that dolphins are always breathing their total freedom of thought, and the author provides insights into how humans can learn from this remarkable trait. The book also invites readers to embark on a journey into understanding the telepathic communication of whales and dolphins. Inclusive in the book is a written meditation which assists you to connect to the external consciousness and release the fear that you have wrapped around yourself for protection.

Overall, this book offers a unique and fascinating perspective on the metaphysics of dolphins, and will appeal to anyone interested in spirituality, and the power of the mind.

Book VII. Decoding The Sacred Alphabet And Numerology

This book offers a myriad of explanations concerning the higher consciousness in relationship to names, places and numbers. "Decoding The Sacred Alphabet & Numerology" by O.M. Kelly (Omni) is a thought-provoking and enlightening read that

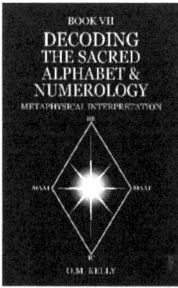

offers a unique perspective on the metaphysical world of letters and numbers.

Omni's insights and teachings are sure to inspire readers to deepen their understanding of the ancient sacred codes to names of places, your name and the sacred alphabet. The author also delves into the practice of metaphysical numerology, which involves using numerical values to interpret personality traits, life paths, and other aspects of a person's life. Omni explains how metaphysical numerology can be used to gain insight into our spiritual path and to better understand our purpose in life. Your ability to decipher the Sacred Alphabet and Numerology codes commonly and constantly presented to you throughout your life, will open opportunities to expand your consciousness and awareness you never thought possible.

Embark on a journey through the myth of Babylon and Shambhala and discover the sacred language that connects us all. Explore Luxor, the Delta Giza Saqqara and Faiyum, and Solomon's Temple, and uncover the mysteries of Akhenaton and Tomb KV-63. Find out how to unravel the threads of your DNA and unlock the ancient knowledge of the Old Aramaic Story of Aladdin and the Lamp. Explore Grecian stories through the Metaphysical language and travel along the Old Silk Road. Discover the Shamanic inheritance of numbers and their meanings, and learn how we rely on numbers to read the hidden language of the universe. Join O.M. Kelly on a journey of self-discovery and uncover the divine language within.

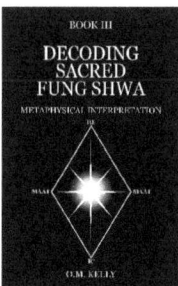

Book VIII. Decoding Sacred Fung Shwa

Introducing "Decoding Sacred Fung Shwa", the revolutionary guide to understanding and harnessing the energy within your home and yourself. In this book, author O.M. Kelly (Omni), has introduced a metaphysical sixth element that takes our understanding of energy to the next level. By incorporating "Your Life Force," we gain deeper insight into the connection between our homes and our emotional well-being. Discover the power of Fung Shwa and learn how to use it to create a balanced and harmonized environment that supports your mind, body, and Soul.

The book explains the meaning of Sacred Fung Shwa to the Shamanistic principles that underpin it. Delve into the metaphysical medicine wheel and explore the elements of life, before moving on to practical applications of Fung Shwa in the home.

Learn how to visualize your home as a collective energy and clear the clutter to enhance its flow. Discover your Astrological colours and how they can be used in Fung Shwa design, from the kitchen to the bedroom and beyond. Explore the compatibility of personal colours in relationships, and discover the power of paintings, pictures, and mirrors to enhance your home's energy.

But Fung Shwa isn't just about the home—we also explore its applications in the office environment and in small retail businesses. Learn how to apply Fung Shwa principles to a clothing store, shoe store, or café, even discover the role of Fung Shwa in money, and to Metaphysical Numerology.

Throughout it all, we focus on the quest of life and how Fung Shwa can help you achieve your goals and live your best life. So what are you waiting for? Dive into the world of Fung Shwa and transform your home, your business, and your life today!

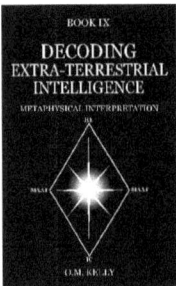

Book IX. Decoding Extra-Terrestrial Intelligence Are you ready to embark on a journey of self-discovery? Look no further than O.M. Kelly's groundbreaking book, Book IX "Decoding Extra-Terrestrial Intelligence". Through metaphysical interpretation, O.M. Kelly (Omni) has unlocked the secrets of the universe and revealed that the key to our next step in human evolution lies within ourselves. This book will show you how to tap into the indelible imprint of holographic importance that is seeded within every human, and unleash the Extra-Terrestrial Intelligence that resides within you. Omni shares her own personal journey of encountering Beings of Light and how it has transformed her understanding of the universe and humanity's place within it.

Omni presents the concept that we all have Extra-Terrestrial Intelligence, and have the ability to tap into the vast knowledge and secrets of the universe. The ancient civilizations left behind clues and teachings about this metaphysical existence and it is up to us to continue to uncover and advance the way we think. Through this journey of life, we can unlock the secrets of our own consciousness and tap into the full potential of our existence. This is a fascinating exploration of the mysteries of the universe and the potential for our own personal evolution.

Readers who are interested in self-transformation through universal truths, Metaphysical exploration for personal growth and a journey of self-discovery would be interested in reading this insightful book on contact with Beings of Light and Extra-terrestrial Intelligence, exploring ancient civilizations and the knowledge they possessed about the universe and the human mind.

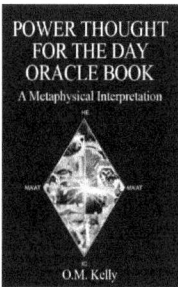

Power Thought for the Day Oracle Book

"Power Thought For The Day Oracle Book" provides insights to assist you on your life path. Through the "Totem" energy of all, the ancient species that have evolved before us, represent an emotional inheritance that we can rely on to sustain the moment. Each species that has evolved on this planet is recorded into our cellular memory. This book with 22 Major Arcana Shamanic Power Animal Totems provides a contemporary metaphysical interpretation symbolic of our evolution. By selecting a page of the book the Shamanic animal will provide an insight in how you are thinking at this moment in time. Through the contemporary Laws of Shamanism (with a metaphysical interpretation), O.M. Kelly (Omni) has produced a book that will assist the "Path of the Initiate" in emotional intelligence when our mind is in the field of doubt. When we become aware of how we are thinking it is a catalyst for transformation. This compact little book is a handy 4 x 7 inches or 10.2 x 17.8 cm to fit into your pocket or handbag.

How to use the book:
Our higher mind has no time; it steps into and works on behalf of the thought of the moment. This book encompasses 22 Major Totem Power representations, symbolic of our evolution. Close your eyes and inhale and exhale a deep breath and relax and allow yourself no thought as you select the right page of the Shamanic animal presented in this book. The right page will always appear for you at the right moment and you will discover how the power animals are working with you for insight into their wisdom. Different power animals come into our lives at various phases offering messages to guide us on our path.

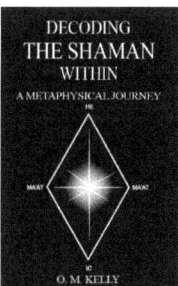

Decoding the Shaman Within

In "Decoding the Shaman Within" international author O.M. Kelly (Omni) shares her Shamanic metaphysical journey. It would be termed a contemporary Shamanic initiation journey; a powerful spiritual enlightenment and transformational voyage of discovering the codes of Metaphysics and the Quest of Life. Through the sacred passage of time Omni discovered the secret codes of the Collective Consciousness (Laws of the Universe) to trek a higher level of consciousness. Throughout

Omni's training to receive the breath of Shamanism, many Elders from other cultures came to Australia and initiated her into their own tribal laws. Most of these Elders were men who arrived on Omni's doorstep uninvited but had received the call from the Universe to pass on their knowledge. Those magnificent people who had also earned their Shamanic experiences, only stayed long enough to give Omni their gift of consciousness and to initiate her into a new Shamanic name, which their tribe had bestowed, and then they disappeared out of Omni's life as quickly as they had come into it.

The Shamanic path in a Metaphysical perspective is the oldest pathway of the tribal law through the evolution of humanity. The Shaman is trained in the ancient language that is instilled in every genetic code that humanity carries within their DNA; you either have the opportunity to open it up and use it, or you just don't bother and choose to ignore it! It is as simple as that!

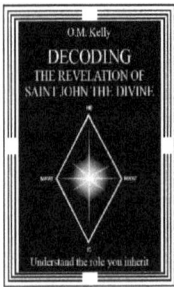

Decoding the Revelation of Saint John the Divine: Understand the role you inherit

The amazing breakthrough book "Decoding the Revelation of Saint John the Divine: Understand the role you inherit", is for anyone with an open, inquiring mind, seeking answers to the surreal descriptions of Earth's final days.

Through years of research O.M. Kelly interprets the cryptology behind the codes of mythology and various religions and has Metaphysically interpreted how the Holy Bible had been written through the original codex of Egyptology. The biblical stories were collected and condensed through the educated minds of that time.

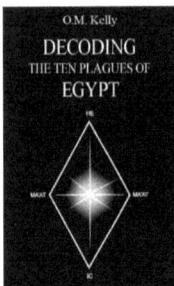

Decoding the Ten Plagues of Egypt

"Decoding the Ten Plagues of Egypt" presents a fresh insight into understanding the hidden structure of the language of how the Bible was written. The reader is introduced to the step by step Metaphysical decoding of the mystifying language, regarding the plagues from the Book of Exodus, Chapters: 7-12 in the Bible.

For the first time in contemporary history the essence of the Book of Exodus and its previously unsolved intriguing language will be revealed to provide deeper knowledge and clearer perception to unlock the significance the Book of Exodus is explaining to us.

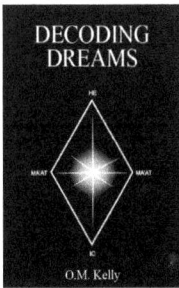

Decoding Dreams

In "Decoding Dreams" international author O.M. Kelly (Omni), introduces a metaphysical interpretation of the dreams we dream. At times, we may believe that dreams allow us to peer into another world. O.M. Kelly provides the codes for us to understand that other world of dreams—or, through the Shamanic Principles, our "Vision Worlds". Dreams are created through your unconscious/higher mind communicating back to you; dreams are reminding you of the lessons that you need to understand regarding yourself. You cannot hear them if your mind is filled with incessant chatter. The ego refuses to conform when it is in control of the moment. Dreams can range from a pleasant dream, which could be a recommendation to add to what you are doing, to a nightmare, which is a wake-up call from your higher self regarding what you are doing to yourself. As you read this book, keep in mind that learning to metaphysically interpret your dreams is a step-by-step process. Areas covered in the book are: Dream Representations (Animal Kingdom and the Human Kingdom), Questions and Answers about Dreams, and Dream Interpretations.

Reprint coming in the near future.